Strength and Muscular Endurance Progress Log

Name:

Date																					
Exercise	Wt	Rep	Wt	Rep	Wt	Rep	Wt	Rep	Wt	Rep	Wt	Rep	Wt	Rep	Wt	Rep	Wt	Rep	Wt	Rep	Wt	Rep

Strength and Muscular Endurance Progress Log

Name:

Exercise	Date																					
	Wt	Rep	Wt	Rep	Wt	Rep	Wt	Rep	Wt	Rep	Wt	Rep	Wt	Rep	Wt	Rep	Wt	Rep	Wt	Rep	Wt	Rep

Weight Training for Life

Eighth Edition

James L. Hesson

Black Hills State University

THOMSON

WADSWORTH

Australia • Brazil • Canada • Mexico • Singapore • Spain • United Kingdom • United States

THOMSON
WADSWORTH

Weight Training for Life, Eighth Edition
James L. Hesson

Executive Editor: Nedah Rose
Assistant Editor: Colin Blake
Technology Project Manager: Donna Kelley
Marketing Manager: Jennifer Somerville
Marketing Assistant: Michele Colella
Marketing Communications Manager: Jessica Perry
Project Manager, Editorial Production: Sandra Craig
Creative Director: Rob Hugel
Art Director: Lee Friedman

Print Buyer: Rebecca Cross
Permissions Editor: Bob Kauser
Production Service: G&S Book Services and Ruth Cottrell
Copy Editor: Betty Duncan
Cover Designer: Carolyn Deacy
Cover Images: Large: © LWA-Dann Tardif/Corbis; inset: © Digital Vision/ Getty Images
Compositor: G&S Book Services
Cover and Text Printer: Quebecor World/Dubuque

Printed in the United States of America
1   2   3   4   5   6   7   09   08   07   06

For more information about our products, contact us at:
Thomson Learning Academic Resource Center
1-800-423-0563
For permission to use material from this text or product, submit a request online at http://www.thomsonrights.com.
Any additional questions about permissions can be submitted by e-mail to thomsonrights@thomson.com.

Thomson Higher Education
10 Davis Drive
Belmont, CA 94002-3098
USA

Library of Congress Control Number: 2005937607
ISBN 0-495-01275-0

Contents

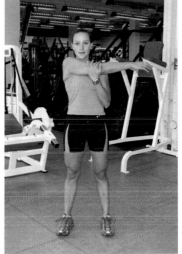

Kristin Dilworth

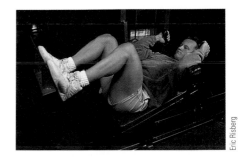
Eric Risberg

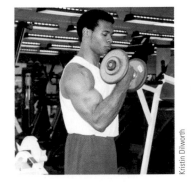

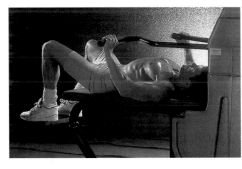

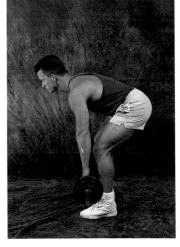

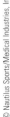

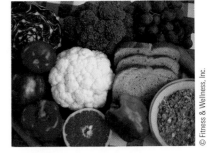

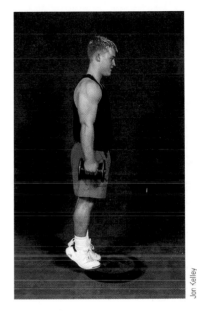

Dedication

To the wind beneath my wings, the creator of all that is, the source of my inspiration and strength, the source of my knowledge and wisdom, the great spirit that lives within all of us, and the great spirit through which we are all joined as one in the endless cycle of life.

To Margie, Jennifer, and David, with love.

To all of the teachers, coaches, friends, and colleagues who have shared their time, energy, and knowledge with me.

To all of my students who have taught me, and who continue to teach me, how to help them learn.

To my parents, Jack and Gladys Hesson, who taught me the basic values and attitudes that have made all other learning and accomplishment possible.

Preface

To the Student

Weight Training for Life has been written to you and for you. Learning about weight training by the trial-and-error method is difficult, embarrassing, and confusing. We hope this book will make learning simple, easy, and fun.

The purpose of this book is to help you build a solid foundation of current knowledge and practice in beginning weight training. All exercise information in this book is consistent with the recommendations of the National Strength and Conditioning Association (NSCA) and the American College of Sports Medicine (ACSM).

This book does not attempt to include everything there is to know about weight training. It is a book for beginners, not for exercise physiologists, strength coaches, or advanced-strength athletes although one chapter is devoted to advanced weight training. This is a book to help you get started *weight training for life*.

To the Instructor

Weight Training for Life has been written to help you and to help your students. It does not attempt to cover everything that you know about weight training, but it does attempt to organize some basic information for you and your students.

One common challenge for most weight training teachers is time. Answer the following questions quickly.

- Do you have enough class time to tell your students all that you wish you could about weight training?

- Are your students always present, on time, and alert for your weight training lectures?

- Do you have other classes to prepare for?

- Are you paid for talking or for helping students learn?

- Do you ever get bored presenting the same beginning weight training information year after year and class after class?

- Have you ever forgotten to mention some basic information that you wanted your students to know?

- Could you be more productive if you didn't have to repeat the same basic information again and again?

- Would your students learn more effectively if they were required to actively seek information?

- Do you have enough class time to lecture and lift?

- Do you teach more than one weight training class?

- Have you ever noticed how the right tool can help you complete a task easier, faster, and better?

This book is a tool that can help you perform your task of teaching weight training. It can make your performance of this task better and, at the same time, easier. A book will never replace you as a teacher because your role is much more important, dynamic, and complex. Your responsibility is to create a stimulating learning environment, to motivate, to provide direction, and to give feedback.

THE MATERIAL IN THIS BOOK CAN BE COVERED IN ANY ORDER YOU CHOOSE. YOU ALSO ARE ENCOURAGED TO ADD OR DELETE ANY MATERIAL YOU WISH. Based on the feedback I have received, there seems to be an infinite variety of ways to help beginners learn about weight training.

This tool can be more effective if we work together. As you use the book, let me know how we can improve it to help you and your students. To those of you who used the first seven editions and sent your suggestions for improvements, you will find most of these in this eighth edition. Thank you for making this revision possible and for making it better.

The **Instructor's Manual** and Test Bank for this book includes

- A philosophy of teaching *Weight Training for Life* based on the author's 42 years of experience.

- An example of a class schedule (what to do each day).

- A quiz for each chapter that you can photocopy and use.

- A final exam that you can photocopy and use.

- An evaluation form for the course and teacher that you can photocopy and use.

- A plan for grading *Weight Training for Life.*
- A form to record points earned by students to determine their course grade.
- An invitation to share your best ideas to improve this book and Instructor's Manual.

Acknowledgments

I would like to thank everyone who helped make this eighth edition possible. Special appreciation is given to the following individuals.

Margie Hesson for serving as a contributing author of this book. Her professional and personal knowledge of exercise and healthy lifestyles brought valuable changes to this new edition. Margie's careful proofreading of the manuscript, in addition to her writing contributions, brought the female perspective to the presentation of the material making this a more balanced text for men and women.

Dr. Larry Tentinger for serving as a contributing author.

Kristin Dilworth, Jon Kelley, and **Eric Risberg** for their excellent photography.

Andre Morrow for all he did to make this book possible. Andre, you are the greatest.

Leslie Araya, Courtney Bennigson, Erik Berger, Blakelee Binning, Sara Brinkley, Grant Conklin, Josh Cooper, Therese Crawford, T. C. Dantzler, Samantha Dompier, Jason Gatson, Sanjuan Jones, Brett McClure, Anna Lissa I. Nool, Chris Parker, Jason Yeske, Jay Adrion, Dave Donat, Jeremy Kinney, Mike Allen, Connie Tyler, Ann Rochelle, Monique Manley, and **Jeni Barraclough** for their time, energy, ideas, encouragement, and patience as models.

Jay Adrion for the use of Jay's Gym for photos.

Werner and **Sharon Hoeger** for being generous and caring to share their knowledge and material with us so that we can share it with you.

Yvonne Adrion for help finishing the eighth edition.

Nautilus and **Universal Gym Equipment, Inc.** for the excellent photographs.

Jennifer Evans for help with digital photography.

Jim Bryant for his friendship and helpful attitude as well as everything he did for me to make the earlier editions of this book possible.

Milton Wilder for his support, encouragement, and friendship. As you know Milton, this book never would have happened without you. Thank you.

Tom Kidd for his early encouragement and support of an extremely thin and weak young boy. He supported my early weight training at a time when weight training was not popular and was not recommended by most coaches. It took a lot of courage to stand up for what you believed to be right, when all of the other coaches thought you were wrong. Scientific research has since proven that you were right and they were wrong.

Jake Geier for teaching me the difference between "producers" and "excusers."

Phil Allsen for his friendship as well as his continuing faith in me and support of my professional and personal development.

Joanne Saliger for making the first seven editions of this book so attractive and functional.

We thank the reviewers of the sixth edition:

James Gustafson, Messiah College

David W. Hunter, Hampton University

Joe Peoples, Coastal Georgia Community College

L. Kristi Sayers, University of Montevallo

William C. Whiting, California State University–Northridge

We thank the reviewers of the seventh edition:

Peter DiLorenzo, Camden County College

Heather Golly, Minot State University

Carol Hirsh, Austin Community College

James J. Scott, Jackson Community College

Steve VanKanegan, University of Southern California

Kristi Ward, Colorado Christian University

And, finally, we thank the reviewers for their valuable comments and contributions to the eighth edition:

Carol Hirsh, Austin Community College

Mac Gillam, Jacksonville State University

Elaine Bryan, Georgia Perimeter College

John McNamara, Temple University

Bethany Larsen, Arizona State University

JLH

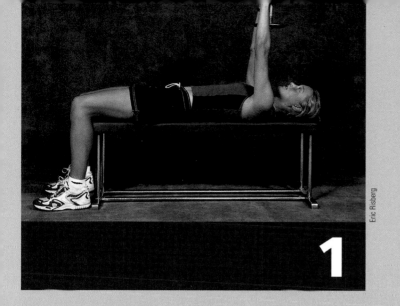
Eric Risberg

1

What, Who, and Why

You have an opportunity to participate in your own creation. The process of your creation did not end with your birth; it continues throughout your life. All of the living cells in your body have a time limit. Millions of your cells die and are replaced every day. In terms of living cells, you are not the same person you were last year, yesterday, an hour ago, or even 5 minutes ago. You are in a continual process of changing, and being re-created. What will you be like tomorrow, next week, or next year?

Your attitude, behavior, and lifestyle choices have a significant impact on who you are and who you will become. Through weight training and healthy eating you start to change your body. You will find, however, that as your body changes, your life begins to change. I challenge you to follow a well-planned weight training program, along with a healthy eating program, for 1 year and see for yourself. After a year of disciplined weight training and healthy eating, you will see such a

dramatic difference, I believe, that you also will believe in *weight training for life.*

What Is Weight Training?

Weight training is a form of **progressive resistance exercise.** Weight can be added to or taken from the total load to arrive at the correct resistance for you for each exercise and each muscle group. Weight training exercises are done for different reasons. The categories of weight trainers discussed next will help you understand why there are so many different kinds of weight training programs.

Who Trains with Weights?

Those who train with weights include Olympic lifters, power lifters, bodybuilders, athletes, medical patients, physical fitness enthusiasts, and weight trainers.

1

Olympic Lifters

Olympic-style weight lifting is a competitive sport. The objective in Olympic-style lifting is to see who can lift the most total weight overhead using two different lifts: the snatch and the clean-and-jerk.

1. The **snatch lift** requires lifting the weight in one continuous movement from the floor to a position in which the weight is overhead and both arms are straight. The lifter may drop below the weight to catch it overhead but must rise to a stationary standing position to complete the lift.

2. In the **clean-and-jerk lift,** the weight must first be brought from the floor to a position on the upper chest and shoulders (clean). Then, from a standing position, the weight is thrust overhead to a straight-arm finish (jerk).

The winner is the individual with the highest total when the snatch and the clean-and-jerk lifts are added together. The competitors are grouped into different body weight classifications so that they are competing against others who are approximately the same size.

Power Lifters

Power lifters compete in three lifts: the **bench press,** the **squat,** and the **dead lift.** The winner is the lifter with the highest total for the three lifts. The competitors are grouped by body weight so that they are competing against other lifters who are approximately the same size.

Bodybuilders

Bodybuilders participate in competition that is more art than sport. Through weight training, they create a living sculpture using the human body as the clay. Bodybuilders attempt to develop maximum **muscular size** while maintaining a balanced appearance (**symmetry**) and a high degree of muscular visibility (**definition**). In this competition, the appearance of the body is most important.

Athletes

Ever since the rehabilitation work of Dr. Thomas DeLorme following World War II, progressive resistance exercise has gradually gained acceptance by the medical profession and the coaching profession. This form of exercise has changed dramatically during the last 50 years. In the 1950s and early 1960s, most coaches told their athletes that they should not lift weights. During the 1970s, lifting became more acceptable for athletes. In the 1980s and 1990s, most coaches required their athletes to lift weights.

Most top-level athletes now use some form of weight training to improve their sports performance and to recover from sports injuries. Because skeletal muscles are responsible for voluntary human movement, athletes who increase the functional ability of their muscular system almost always improve their sports performance.

Recently there has been increased focus on opposing muscle groups. In the early years of weight training to improve athletic performance, much of the emphasis was placed on the muscles that produce the successful sports movements. Although the training did strengthen the desired muscles and improve performance, this type of training often created an imbalance of strength surrounding a joint. Occasionally, the more strongly developed muscles on one side of the joint overpowered and injured the weaker, undeveloped muscles on the other side of the joint. Good weight training programs for athletes now include exercises for balanced development to improve performance and reduce the risk of injury.

Patients

Physicians and physical therapists frequently prescribe progressive resistance exercise as a part of the rehabilitation program for people who have been injured. By training with weights, these patients regain strength, muscle size, and functional ability after an injury.

Physical Fitness Enthusiasts

Many people who exercise for health and physical fitness have discovered the benefits of weight training. The people in this category want to look better, feel better, and be healthier.

Weight training to increase muscle tissue should be an important part of any fat-loss program. Many people have overlooked the benefits of weight training for fat loss because of the attention to calories spent during an exercise session. Although you might spend more calories during an aerobic training session than a weight training session, the increased muscle mass from weight training increases your **metabolic rate.**

You might use as many as 75 calories per day to support the energy needs of 1 pound of muscle tissue. You might use as few as 3 calories per day to support the energy needs of 1 pound of fat tissue. Because muscle is active tissue that burns calories and fat is inactive tissue that stores calories, those who are trying to lose body fat should increase their muscle mass.

Weight Trainers

Anyone who trains with weights could be considered a weight trainer. This book has been written primarily for those who are just beginning to lift weights and for the physical fitness enthusiast, with the hope that if they get off to a good start, they will participate in *weight training for life.*

Who Should Participate in Weight Training?

Everyone who has a muscular system can benefit from a regular program of progressive resistance exercise. Therefore, almost everyone should participate in *weight training for life*—men, women, and children of all ages, including people with disabilities.

Men and Women

The benefits of weight training for men and women include greater strength, increased muscle size, greater muscle endurance, improved appearance, higher self-esteem, and better sports performance. The location and function of the skeletal muscles is the same in men and women. Research during the last three decades has indicated that the weight training principles, methods, programs, and exercises that have worked well for men work equally well for women.

Weight training exercises are the same for men and women. There are no "men's exercises" or "women's exercises." Men and women, however, may choose to develop different muscle groups in different ways, which may affect their selection of exercises. As a result of a well-planned weight training program, men and women alike develop a strong, firm, healthy, attractive appearance.

Is weight training an appropriate activity for girls and women? Absolutely! All women achieve increases in muscular strength when they participate in properly planned weight training programs. Most women, however, do not experience as much of an increase in muscle size as most men on the same training program. This seems to be related to lower levels of the hormone testosterone and a lower number of muscle fibers in women.

Weight training will not make a woman appear masculine or cause a woman to develop any secondary male characteristics such as a deeper voice, facial hair, or thicker body hair. Secondary gender characteristics are caused by hormones. During puberty boys begin producing higher levels of male hormones, which produce the secondary gender characteristics that we associate with males. At puberty girls begin producing higher levels of female hormones, which produce the secondary gender characteristics that we associate with females. This hormone production varies from one person to another.

Although weight training can be beneficial during pregnancy for both mother and baby, there are some cautions. Any kind of exercise during pregnancy should be discussed with your doctor. When weight training is done during pregnancy, you should avoid

- Holding your breath and straining to lift a heavy weight.
- Exercises that include excessive compression of the abdomen.
- Exercises that cause an increase in core body temperature.
- High-intensity exercise.
- Long-duration exercise.
- High-impact exercise.

In other words, exercise during pregnancy should be light to moderate in intensity and duration and regular in frequency.

Children

Children can gain important benefits through a carefully planned and closely supervised weight training program Those who participate in weight training can gain strength, improve their self-image, increase their level of physical fitness, improve their sports performance, and possibly reduce their risk of youth sport injury.

The risk of injury from weight training during participation in a carefully planned and closely supervised weight training program for children is low. The few injuries that have been reported usually have occurred during improperly performed overhead lifts. Contributing factors include too much weight, improper technique, poorly planned programs, and a lack of supervision.

Those responsible for planning and supervising weight training programs for children must be trained and qualified in this area. Each exercise, along with the spotting techniques for that exercise, must be taught and demonstrated correctly. Young weight trainers should not be allowed to train alone without proper adult supervision and a trained spotter. The training area should be clean, bright, attractive, and large

enough for the child to perform each lift safely. Training programs for children should focus on all-around physical development, not just strength training. Strength is only one aspect of physical development.

Children should train with moderate to light weights with which they can handle a fairly high number of repetitions. The National Strength and Conditioning Association recommends 6 to 15 repetitions in each set. This means that a child should not be allowed to lift a weight unless he or she can complete at least 6 correct repetitions using that weight. One-repetition maximum lifts are not recommended for children.

Weight training for children should be on a voluntary basis. If young children are forced to participate in weight training, they are more likely to develop a negative attitude toward this beneficial activity. If they develop a negative attitude, they probably will not participate in *weight training for life*.

After puberty and during adolescence, with the accompanying hormonal changes, children begin to undergo greater physical changes as a result of a weight training program. During this time they should maintain strict exercise form, and close qualified adult supervision is critical. Boys at this age seem to have an overwhelming urge to find out who can lift the most weight one time. Of course, what they often find out is how much they cannot lift one time. The risk of injury is too high.

As young people approach full growth and full physical maturity, weight training can have its most dramatic positive effects on physical performance, appearance, and self-confidence. This is a time when they can handle heavier exercise loads and more intense exercise programs. To maximize safety and progress, however, the emphasis must remain on correct exercise technique. Many young men resort to poor exercise technique to move a heavier weight. This can result in injury. Weight training exercises performed correctly rarely result in injury.

Adults

During the aging process, strength and muscle mass decline. How much of this decrease is a result of aging, and how much is a result of a sedentary lifestyle? Very little of the decline in strength during the adult years is a result of aging. Individuals living in societies that are advanced in technology and automation reveal a much greater loss of strength and mobility as they get older. This is usually the result of inactivity and failure to maintain the muscular system.

Many individuals in the wage-earning adult years think they don't have time for weight training. Weight training actually is an efficient form of exercise. With weight training, a muscle group can be isolated and worked very hard in an extremely short time. A stimulus strong enough to maintain strength or to cause a gain in the strength of a muscle group may be achieved in about a minute with some weight training programs. This can be a greater strength-gain stimulus than the same muscle group would achieve in hours of participating in some adult recreational activities.

All the major muscles in the body can be exercised in 15 to 20 minutes. If a person adheres to this weight training program two or three times each week, it is an investment of 30 to 60 minutes a week. Each week has 168 hours, and you could maintain your strength during your adult years by investing approximately 1 hour per week in weight training. If you have limited time for exercise, weight training is one of the fastest ways to maintain or increase the functioning of your muscular system. It is important for adults to continue *weight training for life.*

Older Adults

At what age should adults stop weight training? Never! Humans should not use age as an excuse to stop weight training. Some physicians advise older adults to stop weight training because of medical problems, but as long as a person has no medical reason to quit, there is no reason to stop weight training at any certain age. Weight training programs, however, do have to be modified with age.

Sometime in their 60s, 70s, 80s, or 90s, most older adults undergo a more rapid decline in physical performance. How much of this decline is a result of the decrease in physical activity that often accompanies retirement or how much relates to a person's deciding that it is time to get old and to act old is difficult to determine. In either case, older adults must maintain their muscular system if they wish to retain their freedom and mobility. Therefore, older adults should participate in *weight training for life.*

People with Disabilities

Many people with disabilities can participate in weight training if they focus on their abilities. There certainly are exercises that they cannot do; however, there are often exercises that they can do. Each person with a disability needs to find out what he or she can do.

Everyone

Weight training is an efficient form of exercise to develop and maintain your muscular system. Though your goals and training programs will change as you progress through life, weight training is a valuable lifetime activity that you should continue. Everyone should participate in some form of *weight training for life.*

Why Weight Training?

The need for exercise has been underscored by the Office of the Surgeon General. The benefits are many and affect all areas of human development—physical, mental, social, emotional, and spiritual.

Surgeon General's Report

The Centers for Disease Control and Prevention (CDC) published *Physical Activity and Health: A Report of the Surgeon General.* One of the findings reported was that "Approximately 15 percent of U. S. adults engage regularly (3 times a week for at least 20 minutes) in vigorous physical activity during leisure time." This means that 85% do not. One of the major conclusions in the report was that "people of all ages, both male and female, benefit from regular physical activity." Also, "significant health benefits can be obtained by including a moderate amount of physical activity on most, if not all, days of the week."

According to the Surgeon General's report, regular physical activity that is performed on most days of the week reduces the risk of developing or dying from some of the leading causes of illness and death in the United States. Regular physical activity improves health by

- Reducing the risk of dying prematurely.
- Reducing the risk of dying prematurely from heart disease.
- Reducing the risk of developing diabetes.
- Reducing the risk of developing high blood pressure.
- Helping to reduce blood pressure in people who have high blood pressure already.
- Reducing the risk of developing colon cancer.
- Reducing feelings of depression and anxiety.
- Helping to control weight.
- Helping to build and maintain healthy bones, muscles, and joints.
- Helping older adults become stronger and better able to move about without falling.
- Promoting psychological well-being.

Regular physical activity should include cardiovascular exercise, resistance exercise (weight training), and flexibility exercise.

Personal Development

Personal development encompasses physical, mental, social, emotional, and spiritual development. Weight training can contribute to all of these areas of personal development.

Physical Development

Weight training makes its most obvious contributions in the area of physical development. All of the following can be improved with a well-planned weight training program:

Muscle strength
Tendon strength
Ligament strength
Bone strength
Muscle size
Muscle tone
Appearance
Posture
Flexibility
Metabolism
Joint stability
Muscle endurance
Power
Sports performance
Lean body mass
Physical fitness
Health

Weight training is a lifetime activity that can help you maintain fitness, reduce body fat, and reduce the risk and rate of injury.

Mental Development

A successful weight training program requires

- Knowledge about how your body functions.
- Knowledge about how your body responds to exercise.
- Knowledge about correct exercise technique.
- Knowledge about which exercises develop which muscles.
- Intelligent exercise program planning.
- Consistent self-discipline to follow your plan.
- Continual analysis of your progress and your plan.
- Insightful, intelligent problem solving.

Social Development

Weight training is an activity that can be done alone, with one training partner, or with a group. Positive social qualities can be developed through weight training with others—among them, sharing, caring, encouraging, and helping. The workouts provide a time to participate with others in an activity that produces positive results for all participants. In contrast to many recreational games, which must result in a winner and a loser, everyone is a winner in weight training.

Weight training provides a common activity in which to participate and a common topic to discuss, as well as a time to be together. It can be an excellent activity for family members or friends because everyone can be together while performing their own individual training program at their own level without interfering with anyone else's progress.

A good weight training program includes the achievement of goals. Sharing your goals with others and helping others achieve their goals is rewarding. A bond often develops among those who do activities together.

Emotional Development

Weight training can help a person release emotional stress and tension. A measurable decrease in neuromuscular tension occurs following a weight training session. It also provides an opportunity to release anger and frustration in a socially acceptable and healthy manner—intense physical activity that is not directed at another person.

Because weight training involves overcoming physical challenges during each training session, some regular participants seem to adopt a more objective and positive approach to other challenges in their lives. This produces greater emotional stability.

Measurable and noticeable changes in physical appearance result from a well-planned weight training program. Increased muscle size or muscle tone, or both, create a firm, shapely appearance for men and women alike. That firm, trim, athletic look can never be achieved by diet alone. Also, posture improves. These physical improvements tend to be accompanied by an enhanced self-image and greater self-esteem. Those who lift weights often look better and feel better about themselves.

Spiritual Development

The spirit refers to the soul or the life force within each living human. It is one of the intangible and invisible things in life that cannot be accurately measured or adequately described. Yet, somehow you know the life force is there. Those who increase the strength of their body and their mind also seem to become stronger in spirit. Stronger people have greater resiliency, a greater life force, a stronger spirit. Many can "talk the talk" but few can "walk the walk." *Weight training for life* can help you become a "can do" person with a strong spirit.

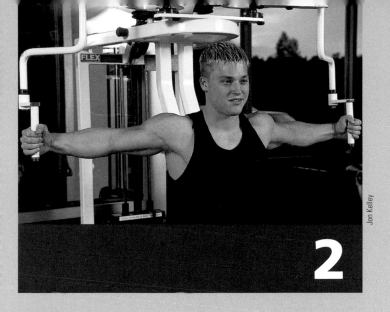
Jon Kelley

2

Frequently Asked Questions

I don't want to get too big, so can I just tone my muscles?

Yes. You can design your training program so you don't get too big. If you use moderate to light resistance (60% to 80% of your 1 repetition maximum) for relatively high repetitions (12 to 15 repetitions) and relatively few sets (1 or 2 sets) of relatively few exercises (1 exercise per muscle group) performed relatively few days per week (2 or 3 days per week), your strength and muscle tone will improve and your muscles will not increase much in size. Actually, a lot of hard work is necessary for most men and women to increase the size of their muscles.

If I build muscle, will it turn to fat when I stop weight training?

No. Muscle tissue and fat tissue are two distinctly different kinds of tissue in the human body, and muscle tissue cannot become fat tissue. If you stop training,

however, you could accumulate more body fat.

Muscle tissue adapts to the demands placed upon it. When you stop training, your muscles will adapt to the new demand. If the new demand is much less than it was before, the muscles will respond by getting smaller and weaker (**atrophy**). If you continue eating the same as you did when you were training hard every day, the extra calories will now be stored as body fat. Even if you manage to stay at the same body weight, you will have less muscle and more fat, leaving you with the outward appearance that your muscles have turned to fat. Because fat tissue is not as dense as muscle tissue, you can expect to gain inches in your body circumference measurements.

To make matters worse, as you lose metabolically active muscle tissue, your ability to use calories is reduced. Muscle cells are active calorie-burning cells. As these calorie-burning cells atrophy, your metabolic rate slows down, and you need even fewer calories than before. You cannot maintain a trim, muscular, shapely appearance by diet alone. Are you beginning to realize the importance of *weight training for life*?

Are nutrition and rest important for weight training progress?

Yes. Weight training workouts provide a stimulus for positive changes to occur in your body, but without adequate nutrition and rest the changes may be slow or may not occur at all. Your weight training workouts could be a waste of time if you do not eat and sleep properly. This is a common problem for high school and college students. For more details, read the Chapter 7 discussion on nutrition and rest.

Will weight training "firm up" a specific part of my body?

Yes. Weight training exercises for a specific body part will firm up weak, sagging muscles and result in a trimmer appearance.

With weight training, can I remove excess body fat from a specific part of my body?

No. The idea of losing body fat from a specific part of your body is known as **spot reduction.** Examples of spot reduction are sit-ups to lose fat from the abdomen and hip extensions to lose fat from the hips. The research on spot reduction indicates that it does not work. Losing body fat from a specific body part requires a reduction in total body fat. This is best accomplished by reducing caloric intake while increasing caloric expenditure.

Is aerobic exercise the best way to lose excess body fat?

No. The best way to lose body fat is a combination of **aerobic exercise, weight training,** and **healthy eating.** Aerobic exercise is a good way to burn calories and develop your cardiovascular system. Weight training is a good way to build muscle tissue, which increases your ability to burn calories and reshape your body. Healthy eating is necessary to avoid excess caloric intake and ensure an adequate supply of the nutrients that you need to rebuild your body. The combination of these three is the best way to lose body fat.

Weight training is an important component of the fat-loss process. The increase in muscle tissue will help with fat loss by building more active muscle tissue that is capable of using calories and by increasing your resting metabolic rate so that you will use more calories even when you are resting. If you want to improve the shape of your body, you need to include *weight training for life*.

What if I don't have time for weight training?

Everyone has 168 hours a week; nobody gets more or less. "Having time" is really about prioritizing. What is most important to you? If you don't have time for weight training, you either have set your weight training goals too high (requiring too much time) or too many things in your life are more important to you. Keep a time log for a week and see where you are spending time, investing time, and wasting time. Many Americans watch television 3 to 4 hours a day but don't have time to exercise.

Does weight training require many hours of training each week?

No. Weight training is an efficient form of exercise. All the major muscle groups in your body can be trained in 15 to 20 minutes, two or three times each week. This is a minimal program, but it may be more than you are doing now and it is certainly better than doing nothing.

The amount of time you need to spend training with weights is related to the goals you set for yourself. Bodybuilders, Olympic lifters, and power lifters do spend many hours each week training with weights; however, that is what they enjoy doing, and they have set some very high goals.

Which supplements and drugs should I take?

None. *Weight Training for Life* is based on healthy moderate exercise, healthy moderate eating, healthy moderate rest, and healthy lifestyle choices. Optimal health is based on moderation, not excess.

Will weight training damage my joints?

No. If done correctly, weight training exercises will increase joint strength. Exercises should be performed in a smooth, continuous manner. Weight training exercises done improperly could damage your joints.

Will weight training make a woman look muscular?

No. Hormones, not weight training, determine if a person appears more masculine or more feminine. Men usually produce much more testosterone than women. The higher levels of testosterone contribute to the secondary characteristics that we generally consider as masculine. Women who participate in weight training develop healthy, shapely, trim female figures.

Will weight training make me muscle bound?

No. If you follow correct weight training principles, weight training will not make you muscle-bound. **Muscle-bound** people have a limited range of joint motion. One weight training principle is to train each muscle through a full range of motion. Each muscle should be exercised from full extension to full contraction. Another principle is that opposing muscles should receive an equal amount of exercise so that the muscles on one side of a joint do not develop more than muscles on the other side. When these principles are followed, flexibility and joint mobility will tend to increase rather than decrease.

The United States has many more **fat-bound** people than muscle-bound people. Their range of motion is limited by an excessive accumulation of stored body fat.

Athletes can become muscle-bound as a result of the unbalanced muscular development resulting from their participation in sports training. When some athletes train with weights to improve their sports performance, they train only those muscles that already are overdeveloped and ignore balanced development. As a consequence, athletes sometimes see weight training as the reason for their muscle-bound condition when their condition actually is the result of a poorly planned weight training program.

Weight trainers can develop a high level of strength and a high level of flexibility, but they have to work on both. A good example of a high level of strength development accompanied by a high level of flexibility is the gymnast.

Will weight training make me slower?

No. I hope this myth is no longer around. Coaches used to tell their athletes not to lift weights because it would make them slower. The research in this area indicates that the opposite is true. Weight training can increase your speed. Muscle contraction is responsible for human movement. If your strength increases more than your body weight, you should be able to move faster. Muscular weakness and excess body fat will make you slower.

Will weight training ruin my coordination?

No. This is another myth that I hope has disappeared. Although some neuromuscular adjustment accompanies an increase in strength, most people make this minor adjustment with no problem. Athletes in a sport in which "touch," or fine motor coordination, is critical might be advised to increase their strength during the off-season and maintain a constant strength level through the competitive season. For weak and untrained individuals, weight training will often improve coordination.

Can I just play sports instead of weight training to gain strength?

No. Most sports do not provide the proper type, intensity, duration, or frequency of exercise to increase strength effectively. Weight training can produce in a short time a strength-gain stimulus that is greater than a muscle would receive from hours of participation in most sports. Many recreational sports injuries are the result of placing an unfit body in a competitive situation. You should gain strength to participate in sports, not participate in sports to gain strength.

Could heavy lifting cause a hernia?

Yes. A hernia, or a rupture in the abdominopelvic cavity, occurs when any of the internal organs is pushed through the wall that surrounds it. If you hold your breath and strain to lift an object that is too heavy, the pressure in the abdominal cavity increases to a high level and could cause a hernia. This happens more often to individuals who do not train on a regular basis. They do not know correct lifting technique or how much they can lift safely. The unfit person moving furniture is a classic example.

It is possible but highly unlikely that a person would incur a hernia during a well-planned weight training program using correct lifting techniques. Correct weight training procedures require that you not hold your breath and strain to lift a weight. Exhaling as you exert force is generally best. In weight training, you should learn about and practice correct lifting mechanics and breathing. These two factors, along with knowing how much weight you can lift safely, should reduce your risk of getting a hernia while you are weight training. Start light and progress slowly. This is a lifetime fitness activity. Hernias occur approximately 20 times less often among weight trainers than among non–weight trainers!

Is weight training for only the young and athletic?

No. Weight training is a healthy lifetime fitness activity for males and females of all ages. Young athletes do use weight training to improve athletic performance, but that is certainly not the only use.

When is a person too old to start weight training?

Never. A person is never too old to start a sensible weight training program. Some people may be too unhealthy but never too old. *Weight training for life* can be beneficial for anyone who has a muscular system to maintain. Each person should have an individualized training program. Your individual goals, training programs, and results will be different, but weight training can be beneficial at any age. Research has shown that individuals who are more than 90 years old gain strength and muscle mass when they begin weight training.

What if I miss a workout?

You will miss a workout—everyone does. Just get back on your training schedule as soon as possible and keep going. A lifetime of exercise is a lifetime of starting over again and again and again. Keep interruptions to a minimum and get back on schedule as soon as possible. Over many years, a few missed workouts will not make much difference. Weight training is a lifetime fitness activity, and the benefits come from years of regular training.

Why should I spend my time and energy lifting weights?

Most people lift weights to improve their appearance, health, and movement. *Weight training for life* can add more life to your years and maybe more years to your life.

Can weight training develop total health-related physical fitness?

Yes. A well-planned **circuit weight training** program can develop all aspects of health-related physical fitness. Total health-related physical fitness involves the development of cardiovascular endurance, healthy body composition, muscular strength, muscular endurance, and flexibility (Table 2.1).

Most weight training programs are designed to develop strength or muscular endurance, but they can be designed to develop all aspects of health-related physical fitness.

	Type of Exercise (What Kind of Exercise?)	Intensity (How Hard?)	Duration (How Long?)	Frequency (How Often?)
Cardiovascular	Large muscle groups Rhythmic Continuous	Exercise at 60–90% of maximum heart rate*	20–60 minutes	3–5 days per week
Body Composition (for Loss of Excess Body Fat)	Large muscle groups Low impact Rhythmic Continuous	Exercise at 60–80% of maximum heart rate*	30–60 minutes	5–7 days per week
Strength	Isotonic exercise Full range of movement Against resistance	70–100% of maximum voluntary contraction[†] 1–10 RM[‡]	1–10 repetitions 1–3 sets	2–3 days per week
Muscular Endurance	Isotonic exercise Full range of movement Against resistance	Low to moderate resistance 50–70% of maximum voluntary contraction[†] 10–20+ RM[‡]	10–20+ repetitions 1 to 3 sets	2–3 days per week
Flexibility	Static stretch	Moderate discomfort	Hold for 10–30 seconds 1–3 times	3–7 days per week

* Estimated maximum heart rate = 220 minus age
[†] Maximum voluntary contraction = one repetition maximum
[‡] Repetition maximum (RM) = The heaviest weight that you can lift for a specific number of repetitions
Developed by Dr. James Hesson, Professor of Biokinetics, Black Hills State University; adapted from NSCA and ACSM Guidelines.

Table 2.1 Exercise Guidelines for Health-Related Physical Fitness

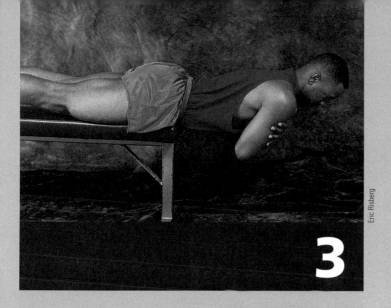

Eric Risberg

3

Muscle Structure and Function

Your body has approximately 600 muscles, making up about 50% of your total body weight. Skeletal muscles account for about 40% of your total body weight, and the other 10% is primarily involuntary muscle of the circulatory and digestive systems. Although muscles vary a great deal in size, shape, arrangement of fibers, and internal characteristics, they all perform the same general function—to provide movement. The importance of muscle tissue cannot be overemphasized. Human movement is made possible by muscle contraction.

Characteristics of Muscle Tissue

Characteristics of muscle tissue include extensibility, elasticity, excitability, and contractility. These four characteristics combine to make muscle tissue a very special kind of tissue. Muscle tissue is responsible for body movement.

Extensibility

Extensibility is the ability of muscle tissue to be stretched. If muscle tissue could not stretch, you would not have the mobility or range of motion you have.

Elasticity

Elasticity is the ability of muscle tissue to return to its normal resting length and shape after being stretched. If muscle tissue did not have elasticity, it would remain at its stretched length.

Excitability

Excitability refers to the ability of muscle tissue to receive a stimulus from the nervous system.

Contractility

Contractility is the quality that really sets muscle tissue apart. When a stimulus is received, muscle tissue can contract.

11

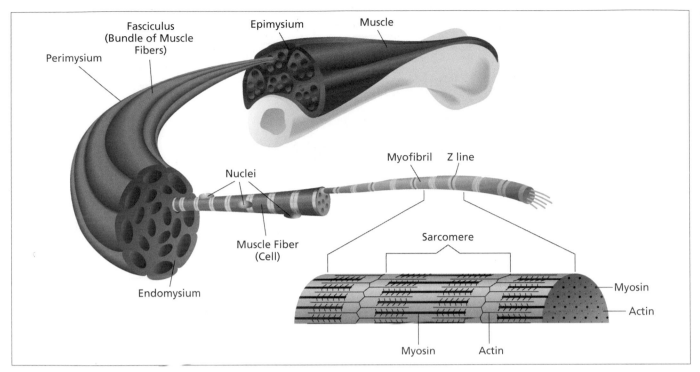

Figure 3.1 Components of skeletal muscle tissue

Types of Muscle Tissue

The types of muscle tissue are skeletal, smooth, and cardiac. Each of these has specific functions.

Skeletal Muscle

The primary focus of this book is the development of **skeletal muscle,** which is attached to the bones of the skeletal system. Skeletal muscle is voluntary muscle—the contraction of skeletal muscle is a result of conscious voluntary control.

Smooth Muscle

Smooth muscle primarily lines hollow internal structures such as blood vessels and the digestive tract. Smooth muscle is involuntary because its contraction and relaxation phases are automatic and not the result of conscious, voluntary control.

Cardiac Muscle

Cardiac muscle is found only in the heart. This type is classified as involuntary because a person cannot consciously contract the muscle tissue of the heart.

The Musculoskeletal System as a Lever System

The human body has three types of levers and six different classifications of freely movable joints. This combination enables a wide variety of human movements, made possible by skeletal muscle tissue pulling on different bones across joints. Some joints, such as the ball-and-socket joint of your shoulder, offer a wide range of movement possibilities. Others, such as the hinge joint of your elbow, are limited to two movements—flexion and extension.

The Structure of Skeletal Muscle

Each of the skeletal muscles has connective tissue running through it and around it. Where this connective tissue attaches a muscle to a bone, it is called a **tendon.** The tendon is continuous with the connective tissue that encloses the muscle tissue.

The connective tissue that encloses skeletal muscle tissue is divided into three categories:

1. Epimysium: connective tissue that surrounds the entire muscle

2. Perimysium: connective tissue that surrounds a bundle of muscle fibers (**fasciculus**)

3. Endomysium: connective tissue that surrounds a muscle fiber

When you stretch a muscle, you stretch connective tissue. The intensity of the stretch has to be sufficient to increase the length of the connective tissue without tearing it.

Inside the muscle are bundles of **muscle fibers** (muscle cells). Skeletal muscle fibers (cells) are generally long and relatively small in diameter. (See Figure 3.1.)

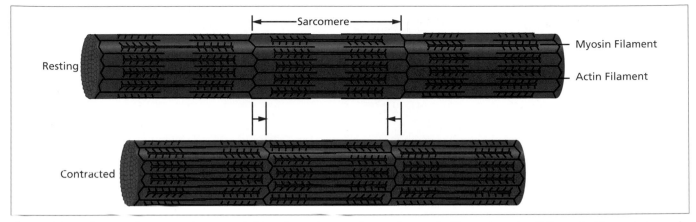

Figure 3.2 During muscle contraction, cross-bridges from the myosin attach to actin filaments and pull the actin filaments toward the center of the sarcomere.

Within each muscle fiber are long, threadlike structures called **myofibrils,** which run lengthwise through the muscle fiber. Each myofibril consists of many **sarcomeres** attached end to end (see Figure 3.1). The sarcomere is the basic contractile unit of skeletal muscle tissue (see Figures 3.1 and 3.2.) Within the sarcomere are **myofilaments.** The thinner myofilaments are called **actin,** and the thicker myofilaments are called **myosin.**

According to the sliding filament theory of muscle contraction, the myosin filaments have cross-bridges that contact the actin filaments. The actin and myosin filaments do not change in length, but the myosin cross-bridges pull the actin filaments toward the center of the sarcomere. Because the actin filaments are attached to the ends of the sarcomere, the sarcomere becomes shorter in length as the actin filaments are pulled toward the center. (See Figures 3.2 and 3.3.)

Muscle Contraction and Exercise Movements

Muscle tissue can contract or relax. Therefore, muscle can pull on bones or stop pulling on bones. Muscle tissue can only pull. It cannot push. In some exercises, an object, such as a barbell, is pushed away from the body. A pushing

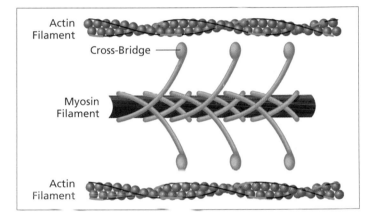

Figure 3.3 At higher magnification, during muscle contraction, cross-bridges from the myosin attach to actin filaments and pull the actin filaments toward the center of the sarcomere.

movement during an exercise is accomplished by muscles pulling on bones and causing joints to extend. All exercises involve muscles pulling on bones across a joint. The movement that takes place depends on the structure of the joint and the position of the muscle attachments involved. (See Figure 3.4.) The types of contraction are isometric, isotonic, concentric, eccentric, and isokinetic.

Isometric Contraction

Iso means "equal" and *metric* refers to "length or measure." Therefore, an **isometric contraction** is one in which the muscle maintains an equal length. This occurs when contracting a muscle and creating a force against an immovable

object. The muscle contracts and tries to shorten but cannot overcome the resistance. An example of an isometric contraction is trying to lift a truck.

Isotonic Contraction

Tonic means "tone or tension." Therefore, an **isotonic contraction** is one in which movement occurs but muscle tension remains about the same. An example is a complete barbell curl. Actually, during barbell and dumbbell exercises, while the external resistance remains constant, the muscle does not maintain constant tone throughout the exercise movement because of the continuous change in its angle of pull on the bone.

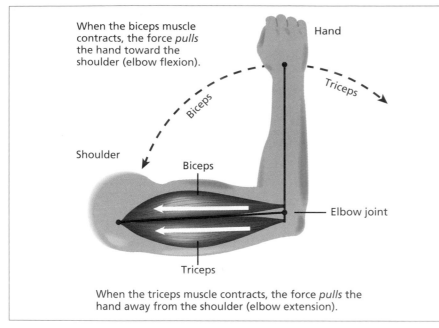

When the biceps muscle contracts, the force *pulls* the hand toward the shoulder (elbow flexion).

Hand

Triceps

Biceps

Shoulder

Biceps

Elbow joint

Triceps

When the triceps muscle contracts, the force *pulls* the hand away from the shoulder (elbow extension).

Figure 3.4 Two muscles showing pulling characteristics

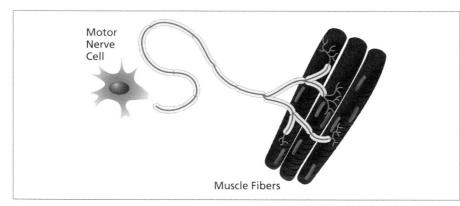

Motor Nerve Cell

Muscle Fibers

Figure 3.5 Motor unit, composed of a motor nerve and muscle fibers

Consequently, another term is **dynamic constant external resistance** (DCER). This is not a new type of training but, rather, an attempt to be more accurate in describing exercise movements against a constant external resistance. DCER indicates that the resistance remains constant, not the muscle tone.

Concentric Contraction or Concentric Muscle Action

A **concentric contraction** is a shortening contraction. The muscle becomes shorter and overcomes the resistance. An example is lifting the weight upward during the barbell curl.

Eccentric Contraction or Eccentric Muscle Action

An **eccentric contraction** is a lengthening contraction. The muscle contracts and tries to shorten but is overcome by the resistance. Eccentric contractions allow you to lower things smoothly and slowly. An example is lowering the weight in a smooth, controlled manner during the barbell curl.

Isokinetic Contraction

Kinetic signifies "motion." Therefore, a true **isokinetic contraction** is a constant-speed contraction. The speed is set on the exercise device so the muscles can contract at 100% of their maximum force throughout the range of motion without causing any acceleration. An example is the leg extension on a Cybex Isokinetic Extremity Testing and Rehabilitation System.

Motor Unit

A **motor nerve** coming from the brain or spinal cord causes a muscle to contract or a gland to secrete. A **motor unit** consists of a single motor nerve and all the muscle fibers to which it sends impulses. Although a motor nerve is connected to many muscle fibers, each muscle fiber is controlled by only one motor nerve. (See Figure 3.5.)

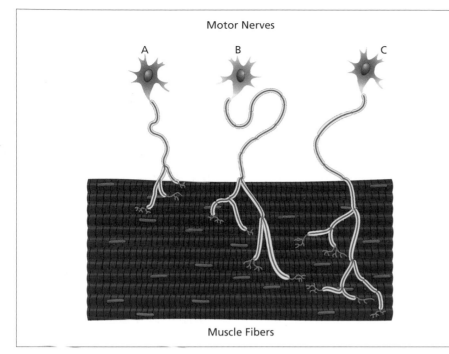

Figure 3.6 Muscle fiber and motor unit recruitment

A motor nerve that is responsible for very fine movement may be connected to very few muscle fibers, such as those responsible for eye movements. A motor nerve responsible for large or heavy human movements may be connected to many muscle fibers, such as those responsible for hip extension.

All-or-None Principle

A muscle fiber contracts completely or not at all. If a stimulus for contraction is below the threshold value, the muscle does not contract. If the stimulus is above the threshold value, the muscle contracts completely. All muscle fibers in a motor unit contract completely or not at all. (See Figure 3.5.)

Recruitment

Each muscle contains hundreds of motor units. The force that a muscle exerts is determined primarily by the size and number of motor units recruited for the task. As an example, refer to Figure 3.6. If a small amount of force is necessary, motor unit A may be used. In this case, 3 muscle fibers contract completely. If a moderate amount of force is required, motor units A and B might both be used. In this case, 7 muscle fibers contract completely. If a maximum force is necessary, all three motor nerves may be activated, and they would stimulate 12 muscle fibers to contract completely, thereby producing more force.

Muscle Atrophy and Hypertrophy

Muscles that are not used will shrink—called **atrophy**—to a size that is adequate for the demands placed upon them. A good example of muscle atrophy occurs with a broken leg or arm that is immobilized in a cast during the bone-healing process. When the cast is removed, that arm or leg is much smaller than the active arm or leg. The same thing happens to people who do not train their muscular system, but both limbs are reduced in size and the process is so gradual that it often goes unnoticed.

The opposite is also generally true: Muscles that are forced to work harder than normal generally increase in size—called **hypertrophy.** This muscle growth is much more visible and more pronounced in men than it is in women. The reason for the greater increase in muscle size in men is related to the hormone testosterone and to a larger number of muscle fibers in a muscle. As your curiosity about muscle structure and function increases, you may want to refer to current human anatomy, human physiology, and exercise physiology textbooks for more detailed information.

Basic Principles of Muscle Development

To develop skeletal muscle tissue, there are three basic principles underlying all weight training progress: specificity, overload, and progression.

Specificity

The principle of **specificity** states that

1. You must exercise the specific muscles you want to develop.

2. You must follow specific exercise guidelines to produce the specific type of change you desire: muscle strength, muscle size, or muscle endurance.

Overload

The **overload** principle is the basis of all training programs. In weight training, the muscle to be developed must be overloaded, or forced to work harder than normal. The overload must be enough to stimulate improvement but not enough to cause injury.

Progression

Once the muscles adapt to a given workload, they are no longer overloaded. The workload must be increased progressively as the muscle adapts to each new demand. The **progression** in workload has to be enough to continue to stimulate improvement but not so much that it causes injury. This is one reason that keeping a written record of each exercise session is important.

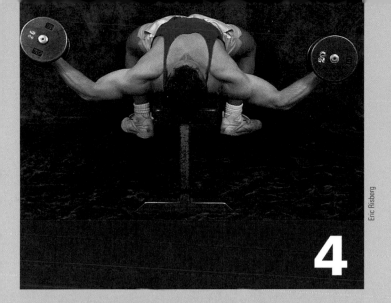

Eric Risberg

4

Warm-Up, Flexibility, and Stretching

The concepts of warm-up, flexibility, and stretching are often intermingled and confused. Each, however, has a separate purpose and meaning.

Warm-Up

The purpose of the warm-up is to gradually and safely prepare your body for more vigorous physical activity. A good warm-up should improve your performance and reduce your risk of injury. The more vigorous your activity is going to be, the more important is your warm-up. Your warm-up can be divided into a general warm-up and a specific warm-up.

General Warm-Up

Your general warm-up should use total body aerobic-type exercises to gradually increase heart rate, blood flow to working muscles, muscle temperature, rate and depth of breathing and to warm the lubricating fluids in your joints. Activities that involve many of the major muscle groups work best. Walking, jogging, and cycling are good for general

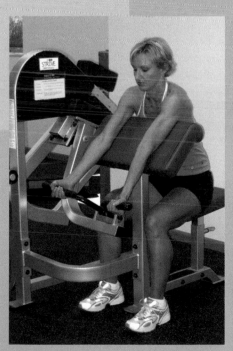 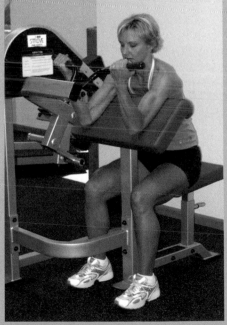

Figure 4.1 Lightweight warm-up sets

Photos James Hesson

warm-up. Activities that require the use of arms and legs at the same time are

even better for a general warm-up for weight training.

17

Start slow and gradually increase your exercise intensity until you begin to sweat. This usually takes about 5 to 10 minutes. Some people like to follow this with a light stretching routine to gently move the joints and muscles through a full range of motion before placing a greater demand on them. Recent research has indicated that vigorous static stretch prior to dynamic activities may have a negative effect on performance.

Specific Warm-Up

Your specific warm-up for weight training should consist of light to moderate warm-up sets for each exercise before progressing to heavier sets. Almost all Olympic lifters, power lifters, bodybuilders, and athletes warm up for heavy weight training exercises using light to moderate resistance to gently stretch and warm the exact muscles and joints that will be used for heavier sets of the same exercise. (See Figure 4.1.) This form of warm-up seems to be beneficial for mental preparation as well as physical preparation to exert greater effort in heavier sets.

Flexibility

Flexibility refers to the range of motion available in a joint. It is specific to each joint and each joint movement. Therefore, a person might be flexible in shoulder joint movements and tight in hip joint movements. An individual also could be flexible in hip joint flexion but tight in hip joint extension.

Correct weight training should increase or maintain flexibility. Proper weight training consists of

1. Exercise through a full range of joint motion in a smooth and continuous manner.

2. A balanced program of exercises for all opposing muscle groups that surround a joint.

Individuals who do not perform any exercise, those who participate in only one sport, and athletes who have trained with weights but have used partial movements or have neglected to develop opposing muscle groups are frequently less flexible than those who train correctly with weights.

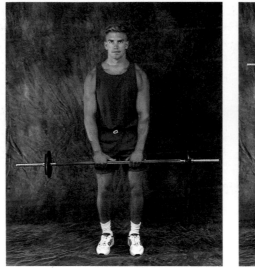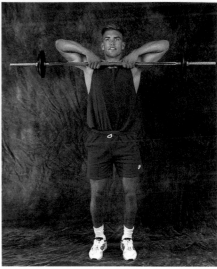

Figure 4.2 Exercising through full range of motion

How much flexibility is enough? There are no absolute measurable standards for healthy flexibility. Some charts report population averages, but in an unfit population how useful is that? In general, a joint should move freely in all of the directions appropriate for that joint.

Is more flexibility better? Not always. There is a trade-off between flexibility and joint stability. If a joint has too much flexibility, it is less stable, and the individual is more prone to dislocation-type injuries. But if a joint has too little flexibility, it is highly stable, but the individual is more likely to incur soft-tissue injuries to the muscles, tendons, and ligaments surrounding the joint.

Weight training can be an ideal exercise to arrive at a healthy amount of flexibility because each joint is moved through a full range of motion and all muscles, tendons, and ligaments that surround and support a joint are strengthened. (See Figure 4.2.) One result of correct weight training should be strong, flexible joints.

Equipment can make a difference. Dumbbells generally allow the greatest range of motion and therefore may contribute more to flexibility. (See Figure 4.3.) The range of motion of some exercise machines is not as great as that of the individual using the machine. If this is the case, the individual will not

increase flexibility when exercising on that machine.

Stretching

Stretching is a type of exercise used to increase flexibility. The range of motion of a joint is usually restricted by the soft tissue surrounding it—muscles, tendons, and ligaments. Therefore, stretching exercises should gently stretch these soft tissues without damaging them or the joint.

Factors Involved in Stretching

The variables involved in stretching include type, intensity, duration, and frequency.

Type

Stretching exercises can be performed in different ways. **Static stretch** is a method of stretching in which the bones of a joint are moved to the point where the soft tissues surrounding the joint restrict further movement. These soft tissues (muscle, tendon, ligament, and joint capsule) are gently stretched and held in this stretched position for a period of time. Six reasons for recommending static stretch are

1. It is an effective way to increase flexibility.

2. The risk of injury is low.

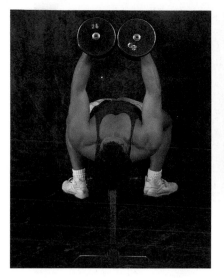 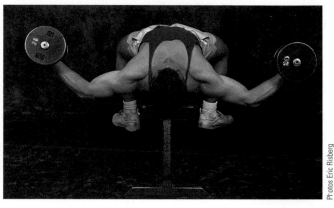

Photos Eric Risberg

Figure 4.3 Using dumbbells to promote range of motion

3. It is easy to learn.

4. You can stretch alone.

5. Static stretch relieves some types of muscle soreness.

6. If done correctly, static stretch does not cause muscle soreness.

Intensity

To be effective in increasing flexibility, the soft connective tissue surrounding a joint should be stretched to about 10% beyond its normal length. Although this is difficult to measure, we have built-in sensors for judging the intensity of a static stretch exercise. When you are stretching at the correct intensity, you will experience moderate discomfort or moderate tension in the tissues being stretched. If you can't feel any stretch, you probably have not gone far enough. If you feel pain, you have gone too far. You should ease into each stretch gradually so you don't get to the pain level.

Duration

When you are performing static stretching exercises, you should hold a static stretch position at an intensity level of moderate tension for 10 to 30 seconds. You should perform each stretching exercise one, two, or three times.

Frequency

To be most effective in increasing flexibility, you should repeat static stretching exercises at least 3 days per week.

Static stretching exercises can be performed up to 7 days per week.

Joints to Stretch

A stretching exercise can be designed for every muscle and every joint in your body, but stretching the major areas— neck, trunk, shoulders, wrists, hips, knees, and ankles—is more practical. Each of these joints is stretched in each major direction that it can move and is held in that position for 10 to 30 seconds. Your weight training instructor can give you additional advice on safe stretching exercises.

Many good stretching exercises have been said to be potentially harmful. Usually, however, it is not the exercise but, instead, the way it is performed that makes it harmful. You always should be careful when stretching so that the exercises produce flexibility and not injury.

When to Stretch

Many people feel better if they stretch their muscles and joints prior to more vigorous exercise such as weight training. This stretching helps prevent exercise injuries and may improve performance.

Some research has indicated that vigorous stretching of cold muscles may be harmful. Therefore, any stretching before warming the muscles should be done carefully. Stretching cold muscles should consist of light, gentle stretching

Stretching Guidelines	
Type	Static stretch
Intensity	Moderate discomfort
Duration	10- to 30-second hold 1–3 repetitions
Frequency	3–7 days per week

Adapted from NSCA and ACSM Guidelines.

exercises designed to loosen the movements of those joints.

Vigorous stretching to increase flexibility should be done only after the muscles and joints have been thoroughly warmed up. One good time to do this type of stretching is immediately after your weight training workout. Another good time to stretch is during the rest between sets.

Weight Room Stretching Routine

The usual reasons people give for not stretching are that "it takes too long" and "I don't have a good place to stretch." This gentle and safe stretch routine on page 20 has been developed to counter those reasons. Although the illustrations show only one side, you should stretch both sides of your body.

If you hold each of these 21 stretch positions for 10 seconds, you can complete this stretch routine in 3½ minutes for a quick, light, easy, warm-up stretch.

Weight Room Stretching Routine

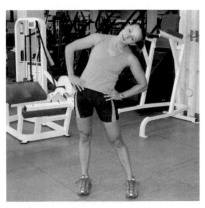

Neck, Trunk, and Hip

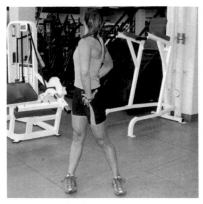

Neck, Trunk, and Hip

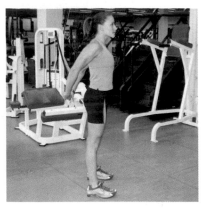

Chest, Shoulders, and Elbows

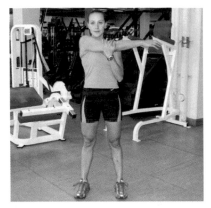

Upper Back and Shoulder

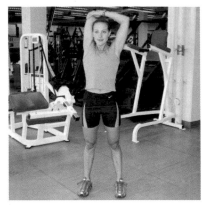

Upper Back and Shoulder

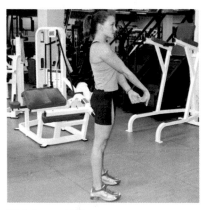

Wrists and Elbows

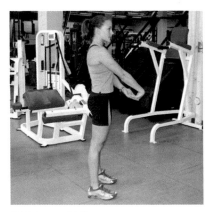

Wrists and Elbows

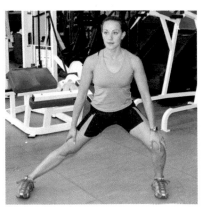

Inside of Thigh

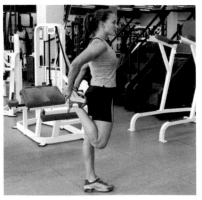

Front of Thigh

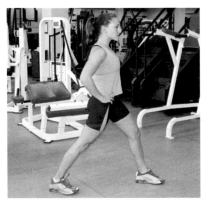

Ankle and Front of Hip

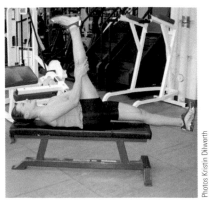

Back of Thigh

Photos Kristin Dilworth

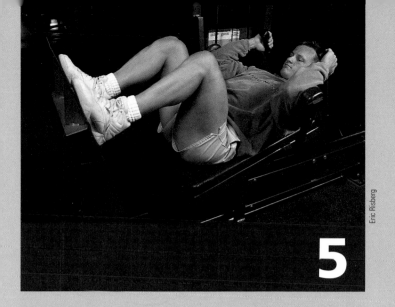

Eric Risberg

5

Safe and Effective Weight Training

For weight training to be safe and effective, there are a number of considerations:

1. Are you healthy enough to begin a weight training program?

2. What clothing should you wear for weight training?

3. Do you know how to perform a weight training exercise correctly?

4. Do you know how to exercise on weight training machines correctly?

5. Should you have a training partner?

6. Do you know what spotting is and how to do it correctly?

7. Do you know the safety guidelines for weight training?

8. Do you know appropriate behavior and weight room etiquette?

You should know all these things before you begin weight training to make it a safe and effective form of exercise for you.

Medical Clearance

Experts recommend that you have a complete physical examination before you start any new exercise program. You should inform your physician that you want to start a weight training program and ask if there is any reason you should not do so. Medical clearance becomes more important as you get older, if you are overweight, or if you have not participated in a physical training program for a long time.

Clothing

Clothing for weight training should be comfortable and allow freedom of movement during all exercises through a complete range of motion. Figure 5.1 illustrates appropriate clothing for weight training. In warm environments, you should wear clothing to keep you cool. In cold environments, you should dress in clothing to keep you warm.

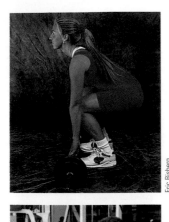

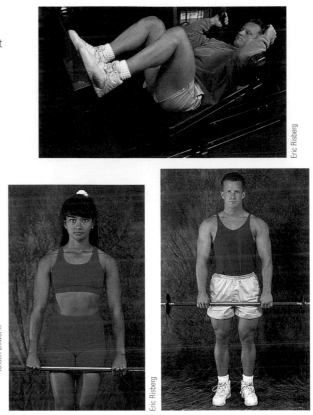

Figure 5.1 Appropriate clothing to wear while weight training

The clothing that you select for weight training should be comfortable, durable, and keep your muscles warm during training. You should feel good about your appearance when you are weight training because, if you don't feel good about yourself during an activity, the tendency is to quit participating. You should wear shoes when training with weights because the weight room has many hard objects you might kick, drop, or step on.

Performing a Weight Training Exercise

The following are factors involved in performing a weight training exercise.

Strict Exercise Form

By maintaining strict exercise form (see Figure 5.2), you will keep the load on the muscles that the exercise was designed to develop. When you do not maintain strict exercise form, you will reduce the load on the muscles that you are trying to develop and increase your risk of injury.

Smooth Movement

Weight training exercises should be performed in a smooth, continuous movement rather than jerky motions. Some exercises are done faster than others, and some involve acceleration, but they should all be smooth. This allows the muscle to apply force to the resistance throughout the full range of motion. The purpose of weight training is to build healthy muscle tissue, not to tear it apart.

Full Range of Motion

Whenever possible and when safe for the joints involved, a muscle should be exercised through a full range of motion (see Figure 5.3). This will result in strength gains throughout the complete range of motion of the muscle. It will also help to improve or maintain flexibility.

Phases of Exercise

Weight training exercises consist of a concentric phase and an eccentric phase.

Concentric Phase

In the **concentric phase** of an exercise, the muscle contraction overcomes the resistance. The muscle shortens as the weight is lifted. For most exercises, this concentric phase should take about 2 seconds.

Eccentric Phase

During the **eccentric phase** of an exercise, the same muscles that lifted the weight will now lower the weight. In this phase, the weight is allowed to overcome the force of muscle contraction. Therefore, even though the muscle is contracting and trying to shorten, it is being lengthened by the pull of the resistance. Eccentric contractions allow you to lower objects in a smooth, controlled manner. Weights should be lowered smoothly and continuously. The eccentric phase of an exercise should take at least as long as the concentric phase (at least 2 seconds) and sometimes up to twice as long (2 to 4 seconds).

Among those who gain the least from a weight training exercise are

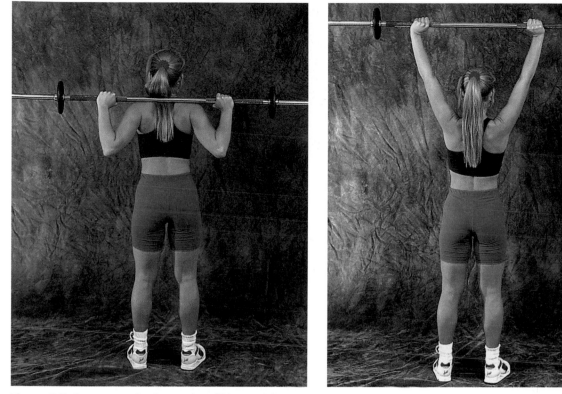

Photos Eric Risberg

Figure 5.2 Proper exercise form when lifting weights

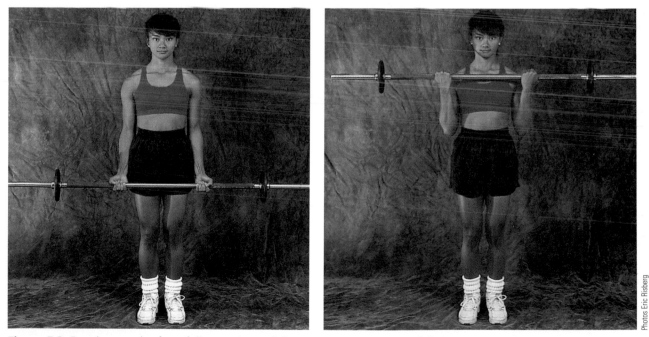

Photos Eric Risberg

Figure 5.3 Exercise muscles from full extension to full contraction and back to full extension

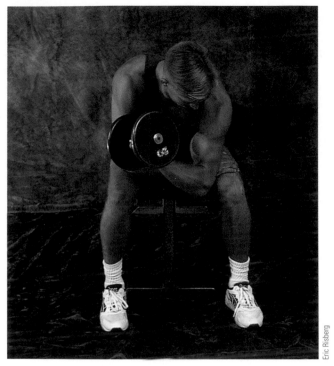

Eric Risberg

Figure 5.4 Focusing full attention on muscles moving the weight

those who throw the weight upward using poor exercise form, incorrect muscle groups, and momentum. Then, once the weight has been lifted, they allow it to drop back to the starting position. Although they may move more weight, their muscles receive less benefit from the exercise and they have a much greater risk of injury.

Breathing

A good general rule for breathing during weight training exercises is to exhale during the greatest exertion—usually the lifting phase of the exercise (concentric phase)—and inhale when lowering the weight (eccentric phase). One exception to this rule may be when performing overhead pressing movements. Some weight trainers are more comfortable inhaling as they press the weight overhead and exhaling as they lower it.

Proper breathing is an important part of correct exercise technique. You should practice proper breathing with lighter weights while you are learning new exercises. With each exercise, you should learn a breathing pattern. There is some room for individual differences and preferences.

If you hold your breath and strain while attempting to lift a heavy weight, this produces a great deal of pressure inside the chest cavity and the abdominal cavity, making it difficult, or even impossible, for the blood in the veins to return to the heart. The sudden high pressure caused by straining to lift a heavy weight while holding your breath could cause dizziness, a blackout, a stroke, a heart attack, or a hernia. Although events such as these are extremely rare in weight trainers, the possibility of their occurring should serve to emphasize the importance of learning to breathe properly during the exercises.

Concentration

Focus your full attention on the muscles that are moving the weight (Figure 5.4). To gain the maximum benefit from each exercise, maintain this concentration on every repetition and throughout every set.

Isolated Intensity

Closely related to concentration and getting the greatest benefit from weight training in the least amount of exercise time is the concept of **isolated intensity.** This means focusing on a muscle or group of muscles that you wish to develop and forcing the muscle to work very hard. As you advance in your muscle training, you will learn how to force a muscle to work to temporary failure. This is beyond the point where you would like to quit and to the point where the muscle cannot perform the task. It is very intense exercise for an isolated group of muscles and is much more effective in producing gains than easier sets that are stopped when they begin to get difficult.

Caution: Working muscles to the point of temporary muscular failure increases the risk of injury and can result in extreme muscle soreness. Progress gradually and carefully to this level of intensity.

Additional Considerations for Machine Exercises

All the guidelines for performing a weight training exercise apply to the use of weight training machines as well. A few additional considerations will make the use of weight machines safe and effective.

Correct Body Position

You should position yourself on the machine so the pivot point of your body—the correct joint for the exercise movement—is lined up with the pivot point of the machine (see Figure 5.5 and Figure 5.6). For example, if you are on an arm curl machine, your elbow joint should be lined up with the pivot point of the arm curl machine. Most machines

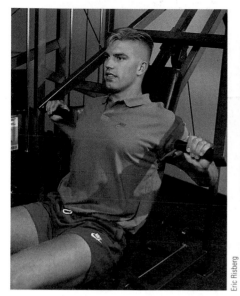

Figure 5.5 Correct body position on machines

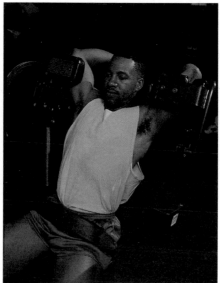

Figure 5.6 Seat belts on training machine

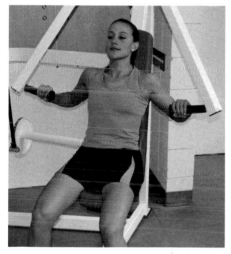

Figure 5.7 Using full range of motion

weight stacks, pulleys, cables, and chains. If you lift the weight stack too quickly, it will gain momentum and could continue upward at the end of the lift, causing the weight stack to bang against the top of the machine. This also may cause the cable or chain to jump off the pulley. At the very least, it will drop with a jerk, dramatically increasing the load on your muscles, tendons, ligaments, and joints.

The weight should be raised and lowered in a smooth, controlled manner. If you allow the weight to drop after lifting it, you may break a plate in the weight stack, the cable, the chain, or one of the pulleys. You can control the speed of movement on weight machines. Lifting the weight usually should take about 2 seconds, and lowering the weight should take 2 to 4 seconds. The weights should return to the weight stack gently and quietly. If you cannot control the speed of the weight, it is too heavy for you at this time. If you decrease the weight and perform the exercise correctly, you will get more benefit and achieve faster gains. Also, your machine will last much longer.

Full Range of Motion

Most weight machines are designed to allow you to lift through the full range of joint motion. If you lift through the full range of motion, you will develop strength, get better muscle development, and maintain a reasonable amount of flexibility. (See Figure 5.7.)

are designed to fit a wide range of body sizes. The adjustments are usually for height. Before you attempt to lift, make sure that you have adjusted the machine for correct body position and that all adjustments are locked in place.

Seat Belts

Several weight training machines have a seat belt to hold you on the machine and in the correct body position (Figure 5.6). Be sure to use the seat belt. It will

make the exercise more effective and safer.

Speed of Movement

Most machines are not designed for speed and power training. Speed and momentum can cause problems for you and the machine. First, you are more likely to injure yourself if you use a fast, jerky motion to lift. Second, you are more likely to damage the machine if you lift too fast. Many machines have

Immediate Repairs

Like all machines, exercise machines have to be maintained properly. If you start to use a machine and find something that has to be tightened or adjusted, do it or report it immediately. Usually it takes only a few turns of a screwdriver or wrench and a few seconds to make it right. But if you ignore it and something breaks, it probably will be much more costly in terms of time and money to get it repaired. Don't misuse weight machines. If you do your

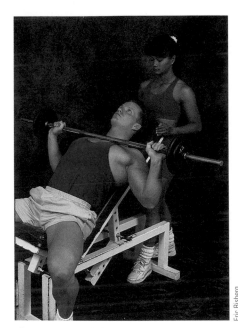

Figure 5.8 Training partner

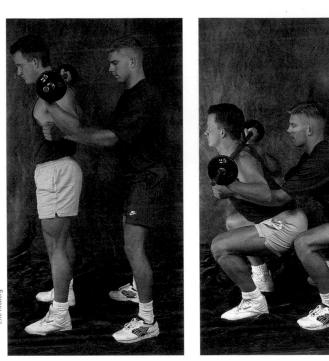

Figure 5.9 Spotting

part to keep them working properly, they will give you years of good lifting.

Cleaning Machines

If many people use the same machines, it is courteous and thoughtful to carry a towel with you during your workout and wipe your perspiration off the machine when you are finished with the exercise. This takes only a second or two and makes it much nicer for the next lifter.

Moving Parts

You should maintain a safe distance from an exercise machine that someone else is using. Keep your hands and fingers away from moving weight stacks, cables, chains, levers, and pulleys.

Training Partner

A good training partner can be your greatest asset (see Figure 5.8.), and a bad training partner can be your greatest liability. A good training partner makes training safer by being alert on hazardous exercises so that you can train to the limit of your capacity with-

out fear of injury. A good training partner is always ready to help you load weights, change weights, and move equipment. A bad training partner lets you do all the work of setting up for exercises. A good training partner offers positive motivation and encouragement. A bad training partner maintains a negative attitude that dampens your enthusiasm. A good training partner is on time for every training session. A bad training partner frequently skips workouts or arrives late.

Even though you can make your best weight training progress with a good training partner, you can make excellent progress training alone. A bad training partner can hinder your weight training progress. If your partner is unwilling or unable to change, you should train alone or find a new training partner. You also should be prepared to listen—you may hear about some of your own faults as a training partner.

Spotting

When lifting weights, especially free weights, you could get pinned under a

weight in some exercises if you could not complete the exercise movement. For safety and to get the maximum benefit from the exercise, you should be spotted on these lifts. A **spotter** is a person who is in a position to help you complete the lift if it becomes necessary (see Figures 5.9 and 5.10).

Communication

Effective communication is the key to effective spotting. Before the lift, the lifter and the spotter should talk briefly. Both the lifter and the spotter should know what exercise will be performed, how many repetitions will be attempted, how much help the lifter expects, if there will be any forced reps or negative reps at the end of the set, if the lifter expects help getting the weight into position (lift-off), and if the lifter expects help guiding the weight back onto a rack at the end of the set. This communication before the lift takes only a few seconds and is time well spent. It significantly increases safety and reduces misunderstandings.

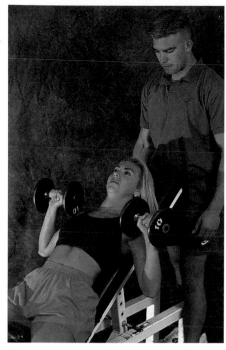

Eric Risberg

Figure 5.10 Stay alert! Give your full attention to spotting.

General Guidelines for Spotters

1. Be sure you are strong enough to help with the weight being attempted. If not, tell the lifter and try to find more help.

2. Know how the lifter expects to be spotted. If you are not sure, ask the lifter before the lift is attempted.

3. Know what signs or signals the lifter will use to communicate during the lift. Know what words and gestures the lifter will use to let you know what to do.

4. Stay alert! Give your full attention to spotting the lift. Do not look away from the lifter. Do not be distracted. Do not carry on a conversation with someone else during the lift.

5. Do not touch the bar during the exercise if the lifter can complete the lift without your help. By doing so, you may decrease the overload stimulus that the lifter needs to make the desired gains.

6. Before the lift, check the bar for balanced loading and secure collars.

7. Move weight plates or anything else near your feet that might cause you to trip or lose your balance.

8. Stay in a proper spotting and lifting position throughout the attempt so that you are ready immediately if help is needed.

9. Do not jerk the bar away from the lifter or throw it off balance. Gently provide the least amount of help needed to complete the lift.

10. Be a responsible spotter. The lifter is depending on you to do the job right.

General Guidelines for Lifters Being Spotted

1. Make sure that the spotter knows what you expect. Don't assume that the spotter can read your mind. If the spotter did not do what you were expecting, it was your fault for getting under the bar without communicating clearly before the lift.

2. Don't quit on a repetition. Even if you cannot complete the repetition by yourself, keep trying, and it should take very little lifting by the spotter to help you complete the lift. *Never* let go of the bar or quit on a lift when the spotter touches the bar.

3. Thank your spotter after each set.

Safety

The following are guidelines for safe weight training.

1. Move carefully and slowly in the weight room. The weight lifting area is not a good place for sudden, unexpected movements. Always be alert for movement around you. Do not back up without checking first. Look where you are going.

2. Stay clear of other lifters and spotters. Avoid collisions with people and equipment.

3. Stay clear of weight machines when someone is lifting or is in position to lift.

4. Fix broken equipment immediately, set it aside, or put a sign on it. Do not attempt to use broken equipment.

5. Make sure you are in a stable position before you attempt a lift.

6. Use collars on all plate-loading equipment such as barbells and dumbbells.

7. Perform all lifts using strict exercise form.

8. Do not hold your breath and strain to lift a weight.

9. Warm up before lifting.

10. Don't lift when you are sick. You are not likely to make much progress, and you expose everyone in the weight room to the same illness.

11. Don't fool around in the weight room. The weight lifting area is no place for practical jokes or wild behavior. Serious injuries can result from thoughtless and foolish behavior during weight training.

12. Do not twist your body, arch your back, or arch your neck while attempting to complete a lift.

13. Lift within your ability. Do not try to lift more weight than you can handle safely.

14. Adjust each machine to put you in the correct lifting position before starting a set.

15. Do not bounce weights off your body or off a weight stack. If you must bounce a weight to lift it, the weight is too heavy.

16. Be careful when loading and unloading barbells that are resting on a rack. If you get too much weight on one end of a barbell, it will flip off the rack. This is a dangerous but common mistake by beginning lifters. Add and remove weight from each end of the bar as evenly as possible, keeping the bar balanced on the rack.

17. Store all weight training equipment properly. Do not leave it lying around on the floor. All dumbbells, barbells, and weight plates should have storage racks where the lifter will put them after completing the exercise.

18. Always control the speed and direction of the lift. If you cannot control the lift, the weight is too heavy. Reduce the weight and perform the lift correctly.

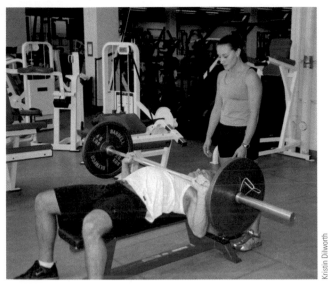

Kristin Dilworth

Figure 5.11 Do not perform a lift in which you could be trapped under the weight unless you have a spotter.

19. Do not perform lifts where you could be trapped under the weight without spotters who know what to do. (See Figure 5.11.)

20. Always be polite, courteous, and helpful in the weight room. This will create a safer and more pleasant training environment for everyone.

Good Behavior in the Weight Room

Weight rooms are often crowded with a lot of people sharing the same space and equipment. You want to be comfortable in the weight room during your workout, and so does everyone else. The following are some guidelines to appropriate behavior in the weight room that will make weight training a more pleasant, productive, and enjoyable experience for everyone.

1. Stay home and get well if you are sick.

2. Carry a clean towel with you and wipe your sweat off of equipment.

3. Don't use profanity, tell offensive jokes, or make rude comments in the weight room.

4. Don't crank up your music so loud that it's annoying to others. If you like loud music when you work out, use headphones.

5. Don't sit on equipment for long rest periods or conversations.

6. Offer to let others work between your sets while you are resting.

7. Ask politely if you can work between sets if someone is using equipment that you need.

8. Take your weight plates off of equipment when you are done. Leave the bar or other equipment unloaded and ready for the next person.

9. Pick up after yourself. Put equipment back in its proper place when you finish with it.

10. Keep the floor clear. Pick up weight plates, dumbbells, bars, and other equipment.

11. Look around and check with others before you change the weight on a bar. If it is still loaded, someone is probably still using it.

12. Don't drop weights, bang weights, or slam dumbbells together. It is disruptive to others and damaging to equipment.

13. Ask politely for a spot if you need one, but make sure you are ready to go. You are asking for someone's valuable workout time.

14. Agree cheerfully to spot if asked. Decline cheerfully and politely if you just can't do it right now.

15. Put weights back on the racks where they belong.

16. Be aware of activity around you so that you don't interfere with someone else who is lifting.

17. Wash your hands immediately after a workout.

18. Keep your hands away from your face during your workout. No matter how clean a weight room appears, whenever you have a large number of people in a relatively small area using the same equipment, viruses and bacteria will be on the bars and other equipment. If your skin is intact, it provides great protection; but if you touch your mouth, nose, ears, or eyes with your hands these viruses and bacteria quickly and easily enter your body.

19. Keep yourself clean. Personal hygiene is important. Don't bring offensive body odor to the weight room. Take a shower, brush your teeth, and wear clean workout clothing.

20. Don't wear strong perfume or cologne to the gym.

21. Stay clear of others when they are exercising.

22. Don't make loud and/or rude noises when lifting.

23. Don't talk on your cell phone in the weight room. Turn it off before you start lifting or leave the room if you get a call.

24. Don't chew gum or tobacco in the weight room.

25. Don't make a mess if you use chalk to dry your hands for lifting. Use a light layer of chalk, just enough to dry your hands. Keep your hands over the chalk container while putting it on your hands. Don't clap your hands together with chalk on them because if you do there is chalk dust in the air and everyone has to breathe it into their lungs.

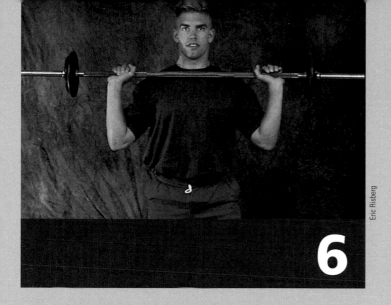

Eric Risberg

6

A Beginning
Weight Training Program

This chapter presents one beginning weight training program to get you started weight training quickly and safely. Some basic exercises are presented for free weights and machines. Which is best for you? You decide. This chapter also includes some basic information on hand grips for barbell exercises, correct body mechanics for lifting a barbell from the floor, some cautions about overtraining, some guidelines for productive training, and a couple of set and rep combinations to get you started *weight training for life*.

Free Weights or Machines?

Which is better, free weights or machines? The following are some of the factors to consider as you decide what is best for you.

Advantages of Machines

1. Safety. The machine supports the weight and controls the direction of

movement, so you don't need a spotter. You should not be able to get trapped under a heavy weight. You can't lose control over the direction of movement. This is an advantage if you will be training alone.

2. Easy to learn and use. Because the machine supports the weight and controls the direction of movement, the exercise movement is easy to learn. On machines it is generally quick and easy to change the resistance. It is quick and easy to move from one exercise machine to the next. This is an advantage if you want to learn the exercise movements quickly and if you want to spend less time weight training.

3. Machine appeal. Some people are just attracted to machines and gadgets. They often believe that anything that is newer must be better. Some of the machines have tried to provide optimal resistance throughout the range of motion of each exercise.

Disadvantages of Machines

1. Cost. Machines are expensive to buy and expensive to maintain.

2. Space. Each machine is usually designed for just one exercise movement, so it is generally necessary to have many machines, each one of which takes up quite a bit of space.

3. Lack of variety. The machine controls the direction of the exercise movement. Most machines are designed for one exercise movement. There is no variety. The movement is always the same.

4. Speed of movement. Most weight training machines are not designed for high-speed movement. Some training programs, especially for athletes, require faster movement speeds.

5. Big and heavy. Most machines are big and heavy, which makes them difficult to move from one place to another. They are not very portable.

6. Accessory muscles. Most machines are designed to develop the prime movers of an exercise movement. The prime movers are the muscles that are primarily responsible for producing the force to move the resistance. However, the muscles that act as synergists and stabilizers are not as necessary on machine exercises.

A muscle acting as a synergist (*syn* = together, *erg* = work) helps the prime movers and helps guide the direction of the movement in barbell and dumbbell exercises. Because the machine guides the direction of the movement, the synergists are not as necessary on machine exercises.

A muscle acting as a stabilizer holds the body in a firm, balanced position during barbell and dumbbell exercises. Most machines have a bench or seat that provides a stable base to work from, so the stabilizing and balancing muscles are typically not as necessary when performing machine exercises.

7. Single-joint exercise. Several machines are designed for single-joint exercise. This is good if you just want to isolate a single-joint movement, but very few normal daily activities are single-joint movements. Most daily activities and sport activities are dynamic and require multiple-joint movements that need to be coordinated.

Advantages of Free Weights (Barbells and Dumbbells)

1. Cost. One barbell with weight plates can work all of the same muscles as a room full of machines, so the total cost is generally less than machines. The cost of maintenance for free weights is also generally far less than the cost of maintaining a room full of weight machines.

2. Variety. Because free weights are free to move in any direction and at any speed, a much greater variety of exercises can be performed with free weights. There is an almost infinite variety of angles and speeds of movement. It is also possible to perform single-joint and multiple-joint exercises with free weights. Free weights allow the performance of dynamic exercises that are similar to daily activities and sport movements.

3. Accessory muscles. The stabilizers, synergists, and prime movers are all developed at the same time in a coordinated manner to control body movement. You develop the ability to balance, coordinate, and control your body and the weight. You automatically learn to use stabilizing and assisting muscles (synergists) to hold your body in the correct exercise position, keep the weight moving along the desired path, and balance your body and the weight as it is moving.

4. Mobility. Free weights are easier to move from one location to another.

5. Fit. Adjustable barbells and dumbbells fit everyone. It is difficult to build a machine to fit everyone. People come in a variety of shapes and sizes: tall and short, wide and narrow, and different arm- and leg-segment lengths. With barbells and dumbbells, your size and shape doesn't matter.

Disadvantages of Free Weights (Barbells and Dumbbells)

1. Safety. Because free weights are free to move in any direction, there is a greater potential for injury. However, if you follow the correct lifting guidelines and the safety guidelines from the previous chapter, lifting with free weights is very safe.

2. Spotter. For some free weight exercises, you do need a spotter. If there is any chance that you could get trapped under a weight, be sure you have a spotter.

3. Ease of learning. Because of the more complex muscle recruitment for balance and coordination, it can take a little longer to learn correct free weight–exercise technique than learning a similar exercise on a machine. More skill is required, but more skill is learned.

4. Ease of changing weights. It takes a little longer to change weight plates on a barbell than to change resistance on machines.

Machines or Free Weights?

You need to consider the advantages and disadvantages and decide what is best for you. You can also do some of each. This doesn't have to be an either–or decision. Both machines and free weight have advantages. What will best meet your needs? What is available to you?

Grips

Your grip on the barbell or exercise machine involves the position of your hands on the bar and the spacing between your hands.

Hand Position

The three basic hand positions are

1. Pronated grip (thumbs toward each other), also referred to as the overhand grip, overgrip, overgrasp, and regular grip. (See Figure 6.1.)

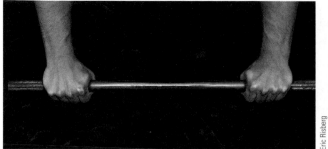

Figure 6.1 Pronated grip (overgrip)

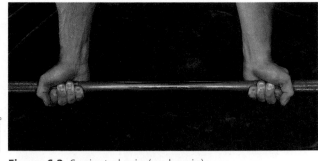

Figure 6.2 Supinated grip (undergrip)

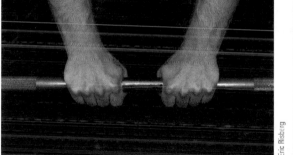

Figure 6.3 Mixed grip

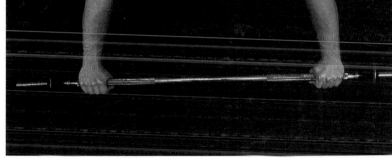

Figure 6.4 Shoulder-width grip

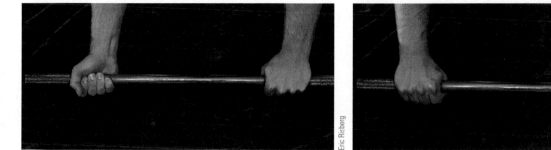

Figure 6.5 Narrow grip

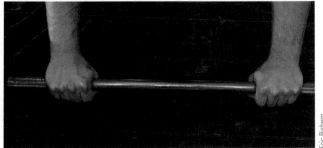

Figure 6.6 Wide grip

2. Supinated grip (thumbs away from each other), also referred to as the underhand grip, undergrip, undergrasp, and reverse grip. (See Figure 6.2.)

3. Mixed grip (one thumb toward the other hand and one thumb away from the other hand), also referred to as the combined grip, alternate grip, and dead lift grip. (See Figure 6.3.)

You should always wrap your thumb around the bar for safety. Performing lifts in which the bar is over your body and your thumbs are not around the bar is risky and is not recommended.

Hand Spacing

The three common distances for hand spacing on the bar are

1. Regular or **normal hand spacing,** in which your hands are placed on the bar approximately shoulder-width apart. (See Figure 6.4.)

2. Narrow grip, which is recommended for some exercises. The hands are closer together than shoulder width, normally 4 to 8 inches apart. (See Figure 6.5.)

3. Wide grip, in which the hands are placed on the bar at a distance wider than shoulder width. (See Figure 6.6.)

When you are learning a new exercise, first try the hand spacing that is recommended or illustrated in the exercise portion of this book. Later, when you have more knowledge and experience, use a lighter weight and experiment with different hand spacing to find the most comfortable and effective hand spacing for you.

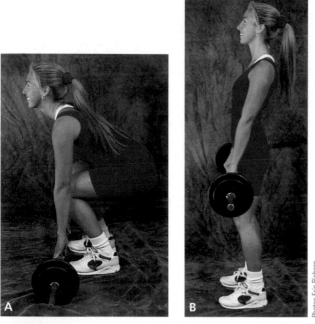

Photos Eric Risberg

Figure 6.7 Always use correct body mechanics when lifting a weight from the floor.

Correct Lifting Technique

When you are lifting a barbell or dumbbells from the floor, always use correct lifting technique. Bend your knees and hips. Grasp the object you are going to lift. Keep the object close to your body. Keep your back flat and straight and lift with your legs. (See Figure 6.7.)

When you are lowering a barbell or dumbbells back to the floor, reverse this procedure. Keep the weight close to your body. Keep your back flat and straight. Bend your knees and hips. Lift and lower objects with your leg muscles, not your back muscles.

Basic Exercises

All the exercises for the beginning program are basic exercises described in the exercise portion of this book. One exercise for each major muscle group or joint action is recommended for beginning weight trainers. Those who are weight training to develop physical fitness usually do not need more than one exercise per body part; however, it is a good idea to occasionally change the exercise you are performing to develop that body part.

Frequency and Resistance

The exercises in Table 6.1 should be performed three times each week with at least 48 hours of rest between training sessions. Start light and progress slowly. If you are just starting a weight training program, you should begin with very light weights and learn to do each exercise with correct technique before you add resistance. Then, gradually add weight, but never at the cost of losing correct lifting technique. Ask your training partner or instructor to watch you perform each lift and compare your technique with the photographs and descriptions in the exercise sections of this book. Have someone videotape your lifts so that you can critique them yourself. Some weight training instructors grade students on correct lifting technique.

Weight training can be one of the most intense forms of exercise that you will ever perform. Muscles can be isolated and worked extremely hard within a minute or two without experiencing total body fatigue. Therefore, beginners tend to **overtrain** and develop extreme delayed-onset muscle soreness during the first few days. This tendency to

overtrain is also a product of the false belief that "If a little is good, more must be better." This is not always the case with weight training. Beginners can easily overtrain the muscles to the point that they cannot recover before the next training session. The result is a decrease in performance and no gain.

The program suggested in this chapter is recommended for healthy young people of high school and college age (approximately 15 to 22 years old) who are near their peak of physical growth and who have been physically active. If you are older or if you have been inactive for a long time, you should progress more slowly. Weight training is a lifetime activity. If you progress slowly and safely, you can avoid the injuries and extreme soreness that result from doing too much too soon.

The First 6 Weeks

Safety, correct exercise technique, and enjoyment are the most important things to learn during the first few weeks of a weight training program. Start with light weights and learn to perform each exercise in your training program correctly. Learn the breathing pattern that works best and develop a habit of breathing correctly during each exercise.

Allow your body to gradually adapt to this new demand. Progress slowly to keep the risk of injury and the muscle soreness to a minimum. Learn to concentrate on the muscles being developed during each repetition of each exercise.

Learn to enjoy each weight training session. Normal humans seek pleasure and avoid pain. Make your weight training time a pleasure. The following are three options for sets and repetitions for your first 6 weeks of training.

Set and Rep Option 1

Weeks 1 and 2 (1 × 20)
Weeks 3 and 4 (1 × 20) (1 × 10)
Weeks 5 and 6 (1 × 20) (1 × 10) (1 × 5)

Exercise Description	Free Weights	Machines
Chest (Chapter 8)	Barbell bench press	Prone or seated chest press
Back (Chapter 9)	One dumbbell rowing	Seated or low pulley rowing
Shoulders (Chapter 10)	Overhead press	Seated overhead press
Arms (Chapter 11)	Barbell curl	Arm curl
Thighs (Chapter 12)	Squat	Leg press
Calves (Chapter 12)	One dumbbell calf raise	Calf raise or calf press
Abdominals (Chapter 13)	Abdominal crunches	Ab machine crunches
Back Extension (Chapter 13)	Back extension	Back extension

Table 6.1 Recommended Exercises for Beginners

Weeks 1 and 2 (1 × 20)

For the first 2 weeks (6 exercise sessions), perform each exercise once (1 set), completing 20 exercise movements (20 repetitions) in that set.

Example: Bench press: 1 set of 20 repetitions (1 × 20)

If you complete all 20 repetitions while maintaining correct exercise technique, you may increase the resistance for your next training session. If a weight feels very light and the repetitions are very easy, you could make a large increase in the weight for your next training session. If a weight feels moderately difficult, you should make a small increase for your next training session. By the end of 2 weeks (6 training sessions), you should be training with a weight that makes it challenging for you to complete 20 repetitions while maintaining correct lifting technique.

If you complete at least 15 repetitions but fewer than 20, use the same resistance for your next training session. During the next training session try to increase the number of repetitions that you can complete with that same resistance. If you complete less than 15 repetitions, reduce the resistance for your next training session.

Any time that you begin to use incorrect lifting technique to move the weight, stop, use a lighter weight, and repeat the set or schedule a lighter weight for your next training session.

Don't sacrifice proper exercise form to complete repetitions. When you can no longer perform repetitions correctly, stop the set and record the number of repetitions that you performed correctly. See the progress log at the end of this chapter.

Why only one set? One set of each exercise allows enough time to

- Locate the equipment for each exercise.
- Become familiar with the weight room.
- Not feel rushed.
- Look around.
- Change clothes before and after.
- Ask questions.
- Receive instruction.
- Take care of administrative details.
- Meet people.
- Find a training partner.
- Find spotters.
- Enjoy your training session.

Why 20 repetitions? Twenty repetitions is enough continuous repetitions to

- Train muscles to new movement patterns.
- Learn correct exercise technique.
- Focus on technique not resistance.
- Keep the resistance relatively low for safety.

- Keep the training intensity relatively low.
- Begin to develop muscle endurance.
- Feel what it is like to train for muscle endurance.
- Feel a slight burning and fatigue sensation in the working muscles to help you identify which muscles are moving the weight and being developed by each exercise.
- Learn to connect the muscles and the exercises more quickly.
- Feel a muscle pump in the working muscles.
- Feel a slight delayed onset muscle soreness in the muscles that were exercised, enough to feel like your muscles were exercised but not enough to turn you off to weight training exercise.
- Reduce the risk of injury during the first 2 weeks because the resistance is kept low.
- Keep the total training volume low for the first 2 weeks.

Weeks 3 and 4 (1 × 20) (1 × 10)

During the next 2 weeks (6 training sessions), perform 1 set of 20 repetitions (1 × 20), followed by 1 set of 10 repetitions (1 × 10). Keep trying to find a weight that is challenging for 20 repetitions on the first set.

After resting 1 or 2 minutes, perform 1 set of 10 repetitions. Each time that you complete 10 repetitions in the second set, schedule a heavier weight for the next training session. Following this procedure, gradually work toward the heaviest weight that you can lift 20 times in the first set and the heaviest weight that you can lift 10 times in the second set while maintaining strict exercise form. If you cannot complete at least 8 repetitions in the second set, reduce the resistance for your next training session.

Why (1 × 20)?

■ To continue developing muscle endurance

■ To warm up for a heavier weight in the second set

■ To continue working on correct exercise technique

Why (1 × 10)?

■ To be able to increase the resistance in the second set

■ To increase training volume (2 sets instead of 1, 30 reps instead of 20)

■ To learn about rest between sets

■ To learn what training for muscle hypertrophy or body shaping feels like

Weeks 5 and 6 (1 × 20) (1 × 10) (1 × 5)

During weeks 5 and 6 (the next 6 workouts), perform 1 set of 20 repetitions (1 × 20) in your first set, 1 set of 10 repetitions (1 × 10) in your second set, and 1 set of 5 repetitions (1 × 5) in your third set. Continue to search safely for the heaviest weight that you can handle in each set. If you complete 5 good repetitions in the third set, schedule a heavier weight for your next training session. If you complete at least 3 repetitions in your third set, keep that weight and try to increase your reps. If you cannot complete at least 3 good repetitions, reduce the weight for your next training session.

Why (1 × 20)?

■ To continue developing muscle endurance

■ To warm up for the heavier weights in the next 2 sets

■ To continue working on correct exercise technique

Why (1 × 10)?

■ To be able to increase the resistance in your second set

■ To continue working on muscle hypertrophy or body shaping

Why (1 × 5)?

■ To be able to increase the resistance in your third set

■ To increase your training volume (3 sets instead of 2, 35 reps instead of 30)

■ To learn what training for muscle strength feels like (heavier weight, lower reps)

■ To develop more strength

■ To learn to handle heavier weights safely

At the end of this 6-week program, most people can safely test for strength and muscle endurance.

Set and Rep Option 2

Weeks 1 and 2 (1 × 20): muscle endurance
Weeks 3 and 4 (2 × 10): muscle hypertrophy and body shaping
Weeks 5 and 6 (3 × 5): muscle strength

With this set and rep option, the training volume (sets × reps) stays about the same, but the resistance increases as you move to fewer reps per set. One advantage of this option is that you have an opportunity to feel what it is like to train for muscle endurance, muscle hypertrophy, and muscle strength before you set your own training goals and plan your own training program. As with all training, you need to use good judgment. Not everyone is comfortable or capable of progressing to heavy weight and low reps this quickly, but some are and there is no reason to hold back those who are capable. Always use good judgment, train safe, and train smart.

Set and Rep Option 3

Weeks 1 and 2 (1 × 10)
Weeks 3 and 4 (2 × 10)
Weeks 5 and 6 (3 × 10)

With this set and rep option, one advantage is that the resistance remains about the same and the volume of exercise (sets × reps) increases every 2 weeks. One of the disadvantages of this option is that you never get to feel the burn and fatigue of 20 reps or the resistance of 5 reps; therefore, you don't know what it feels like to train for muscle endurance or for muscle strength.

Guidelines for Productive Training

After this first 6 weeks of training, you should have had time to develop a good foundation of total body strength and time to finish reading this book, so you are able to plan your own weight training programs based on goals that you have set for yourself. You should be able to plan a method of record keeping and measuring your progress toward your goals. Some overall guidelines are

1. Perform each repetition with correct technique and complete concentration.

2. Make gradual increases in resistance as you are able.

3. Complete each scheduled training session. Form the habit of never skipping a scheduled training session.

4. Maintain a positive attitude. Enjoy each training session. Have fun. Make this the most fun part of your day.

5. Eat right. Healthy eating is critical to optimal weight training progress.

6. Get enough rest. Weight training serves only as a stimulus for positive changes to take place in your body. The changes are biological adaptations that actually take place between exercise sessions. Without adequate nutrition and rest, it is difficult for these positive changes to take place.

7. Stay healthy. You may not normally think of this as a choice, but it is. Your health is closely related to your lifestyle. Make healthy choices.

STRENGTH AND MUSCULAR ENDURANCE PROGRESS LOG (FREE WEIGHTS)

Name

Date																																
Exercise	Wt	Rep	Wt	Rep	Wt	Rep	Wt	Rep	Wt	Rep	Wt	Rep	Wt	Rep	Wt	Rep	Wt	Rep	Wt	Rep	Wt	Rep	Wt	Rep	Wt	Rep	Wt	Rep	Wt	Rep	Wt	Rep
Barbell Bench Press																																
One Dumbbell Rowing																																
Overhead Press																																
Barbell Curl																																
Barbell or Dumbbell Squat																																
One Dumbbell Calf Raise																																
Abdominal Crunches																																
Back Extension																																

STRENGTH AND MUSCULAR ENDURANCE PROGRESS LOG

Name																										
Date																										
Exercise	Wt	Rep	Wt	Rep	Wt	Rep	Wt	Rep	Wt	Rep	Wt	Rep	Wt	Rep	Wt	Rep	Wt	Rep	Wt	Rep	Wt	Rep	Wt	Rep	Wt	Rep

STRENGTH AND MUSCULAR ENDURANCE PROGRESS LOG (MACHINES)

Name

Date																															
Exercise	Wt	Rep	Wt	Rep	Wt	Rep	Wt	Rep	Wt	Rep	Wt	Rep	Wt	Rep	Wt	Rep	Wt	Rep	Wt	Rep	Wt	Rep	Wt	Rep	Wt	Rep	Wt	Rep	Wt	Rep	Wt	Rep
Chest Press																																
Rowing																																
Overhead Press																																
Arm Curl																																
Leg Press																																
Calf Press																																
Ab Machine Crunches																																
Back Extension																																

STRENGTH AND MUSCULAR ENDURANCE PROGRESS LOG

Name

Date

Exercise	Wt	Rep	W/t	Rep	Wt	Rep	Wt	Rep	Wt	Rep	Wt	Rep	Wt	Rep	Wt	Rep	Wt	Rep	Wt	Rep	Wt	Rep

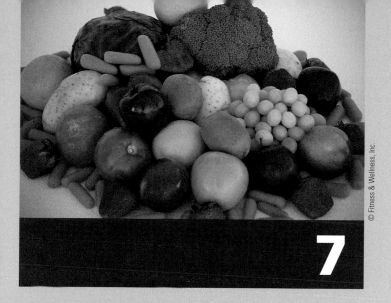
© Fitness & Wellness, Inc.

7

Nutrition, Rest, and Drugs

Nutrition, rest, and drugs can all have a significant influence on your response to a weight training exercise program.

Nutrition

This section includes a brief description of essential nutrients, tools for healthy eating, guidelines for healthy body composition, and a brief discussion of supplements.

Essential Nutrients

Healthy dietary habits will help you get the maximum benefit from your weight training program and will help you maintain a higher level of health throughout your life. The **essential nutrients** your body needs to function properly have been classified into six categories:

- Water
- Minerals
- Vitamins
- Carbohydrates
- Fats
- Protein

Water, minerals, and vitamins do not contain calories or supply energy, but they are necessary for the release of energy and other important aspects of chemical changes in your body. Carbohydrates, fats, and proteins supply energy, which is measured in **calories.** (See Table 7.1.)

The essential nutrients provide the chemicals necessary for your body to

- Produce energy.
- Grow and develop new tissue.
- Repair damaged tissue.
- Conduct nerve impulses.
- Regulate life processes.

Water

Water does not contain calories or vitamins, yet it is essential for your body to function properly. Approximately 60% of your body weight is water. Water mole-

	Functions	Sources
Water	Carries nutrients and removes waste; dissolves amino acids, glucose, and minerals; cleans body by removing toxins; regulates body temperature	Liquids, fruits, and vegetables
Proteins	Help build new tissue to keep hair, skin, and eyesight healthy; build antibodies, enzymes, hormones, and other compounds; provide fuel for body	Meat, poultry, fish, eggs, beans, nuts, cheese, vegetables, some fruits, pastas, breads, cereal, tofu, and rice
Carbohydrates	Provide energy	Grains, cereal, pasta, some fruits and vegetables, nuts, milk, and sugars
Fats		
Saturated fats	Provide energy; trigger production of cholesterol and LDL	Red meat, dairy products, egg yolks, and coconut and palm oils; shortening; stick margarine; commercial baked goods
Unsaturated fats	Also provide energy but trigger more HDL production and less cholesterol and LDL production	Some fish; avocados; olive, canola, and peanut oils
Vitamins	Facilitate use of other nutrients; involved in regulating growth, maintaining tissue, and manufacturing blood cells, hormones, and other body components	Fruits, vegetables, grains, some meat and dairy products
Minerals	Help build bones and teeth; aid in muscle function and nervous system activity; assist in various body functions including growth and energy production	Many foods

Table 7.1 Essential Nutrients

cules make up about 85% of your blood, 70% of your muscles, and 75% of your brain.

Water comes from a variety of sources. In addition to the water that you drink, you get some water from the food that you eat. For example, some fruits, such as melons, are as much as 80% water.

When you are thirsty, your body is asking for water, H_2O molecules, yet thirst is not always an accurate indicator of your need for water. In fact, thirst may be a warning sign of dehydration. Don't wait until you are thirsty to consume water. An average-sized person with an average activity level generally needs to drink about eight to ten glasses of water a day.

Factors including your size, activity level, environment, and diet affect your need for water intake. If you do not take in enough water, your body cannot continue to function properly. Your health and performance will suffer.

Minerals

Minerals are inorganic substances that are necessary for some of the chemical activities that go on continuously in your body. Minerals are essential in regulating body functions such as muscle contraction, protein synthesis, and heart function.

The **major minerals** that your body needs include calcium, phosphorous, magnesium, sodium, potassium, and chloride. Because these minerals are found in a variety of foods, mineral deficiencies are not common in people who are eating a balanced diet. One possible exception is calcium. In a Na-

tional Academy of Sciences study, 80% of the women over age 18 who were surveyed consumed too little calcium. Adequate calcium intake during childhood and adolescence is vital for strong, healthy bones. A calcium deficiency can contribute to osteoporosis (a thinning of the bones).

When your nutritional requirements are met, bones respond to weight training in a positive way by becoming stronger. The benefits occur only to the bones involved in the activity. For example, if you use your arms to lift weights, the bones in your arms become stronger along with the muscles and connective tissue.

Trace minerals are those you need in smaller amounts. They include minerals such as iron, zinc, copper, fluoride, and selenium. Even though

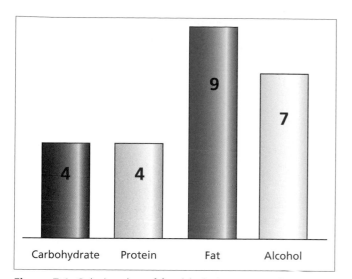

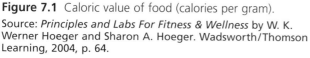

Figure 7.1 Caloric value of food (calories per gram).

Source: *Principles and Labs For Fitness & Wellness* by W. K. Werner Hoeger and Sharon A. Hoeger. Wadsworth/Thomson Learning, 2004, p. 64.

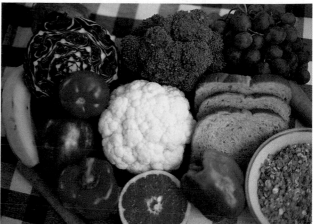

A balanced diet is essential for maintaining good health.

your body only requires trace minerals in small amounts, they are still essential for your health. Some women do not get enough iron. A survey by the U.S. Department of Agriculture (USDA) discovered that many women between the ages of 19 and 50 only get about 60% of the iron they need each day. This can lead to too few red blood cells in the bloodstream, a condition known as iron deficiency anemia. The safest way to prevent mineral deficiencies is to eat a balanced diet.

Vitamins

Vitamins are organic substances that are necessary for some of the continuous chemical activity in your body. Vitamins do not contain calories and therefore do not directly supply energy. However, they are essential to release the energy stored in carbohydrates, fats, and proteins. They are also necessary for building tissue and controlling the body's use of food.

Your body needs 13 vitamins. The two major categories of vitamins are

- fat-soluble vitamins (A, D, E, K)
- water-soluble vitamins (C and the eight B-complex vitamins)

Excess water-soluble vitamins normally are excreted in the urine. Because the body can store fat-soluble vitamins,

you can take in too much of these. A toxic effect can result when certain vitamins are taken in excess amounts. Getting your vitamins from a balanced diet of nutrient-dense foods instead of vitamin supplements is generally healthier.

Carbohydrates

Carbohydrates are a major source of energy containing about 4 calories per gram (see Figure 7.1). Excess carbohydrates that are not used for energy or other chemical reactions are stored as body fat.

Simple carbohydrates, sometimes referred to as simple sugars, are often high in calories but low in vitamins and minerals. Cookies, soft drinks, and candy are examples of simple carbohydrates.

Complex carbohydrates provide your body with many of the valuable nutrients needed to keep you healthy. Breads, fruits, vegetables, rice, pasta, and cereals are examples of complex carbohydrates.

Fiber, another complex carbohydrate, is the indigestible material in food. Nutritionists encourage people to add fiber to their diets because of the proven health benefits such as lower blood cholesterol levels and proper digestion and elimination. Good sources of fiber are wheat and corn bran, leafy

greens, and the skins of fruits and root vegetables.

Fats

Dietary fats, or **lipids,** are the most concentrated source of energy at 9 calories per gram. That is more than twice the calories in a gram of carbohydrate or protein. Excess dietary fats that are not used for energy or other chemical processes are stored as body fat.

Fats are essential components of cell walls and nerve fibers. They are involved in absorbing and transporting fat-soluble vitamins, supporting and cushioning organs, and insulating your body. Fats provide up to 70% of your energy needs during low-level physical activity.

Although some fat in your diet is beneficial, it is possible to consume too much. Excess fat in your diet contributes to obesity, high blood pressure, heart disease, diabetes, and some cancers.

Dietary fats come in several forms. Some forms of fat contribute to health while other forms can contribute to disease. **Unsaturated fats,** including **monounsaturated fats, polyunsaturated fats,** and **omega-3 fatty acids** are generally considered "good fats" due to their associated health benefits. Most of your dietary fat calories should come from unsaturated fats. Sources of

Fat	Sources	What It Does
Saturated Fats	Red meat, dairy products, egg yolks, coconut and palm oils	Provides energy; triggers production of harmful LDL cholesterol
Unsaturated Fats		
Monounsaturated Fats	Some fish; avocados; olive, canola, and peanut oils	Also provides energy, but triggers more HDL production and less LDL cholesterol production
Polyunsaturated Fats	Some fish; corn, sesame, soybean, and safflower oils	Similar to monounsaturated fats
Omega-3 Fatty Acids	Fish (tuna, salmon, sardines, bluefish, trout)	Reduce the risk of clotting by thinning the blood; may protect against hardening of arteries
Trans fats	Shortening, stick margarine, baked goods	Promote production of harmful LDL cholesterol
Triglycerides	Any food that contains fat	Not fully broken down by the liver, they have effects similar to those of saturated fats

Source: *An Invitation To Health,* 10th ed., by Dianne Hales. Wadsworth/Thomson Learning, 2003, p. 150.

Table 7.2 Forms of Dietary Fats

unsaturated fats include fish, avocados, corn, olive oil, canola oil, corn oil, and other vegetable oils.

Trans fats are an altered form of unsaturated fat. Because of the link between heart disease risk and high dietary intakes of trans fats, they need to be limited in a healthy diet. Trans fats are found in foods such as baked goods, fried foods, and some margarine products.

Saturated fats require special mention because of the associated risk for cardiovascular disease. Saturated fats contribute to an increase in blood cholesterol levels. Blood cholesterol level is affected more by the consumption of dietary fat than by the consumption of cholesterol. Elevated blood cholesterol is a major risk factor for heart disease. Less than 7 to 10% of your total daily caloric intake should come from saturated fats. Foods high in saturated fats include red meat, whole milk, butter, cheese, ice cream, egg yolks, animal fat, palm oil, and coconut oil. Keep your intake of saturated fats low. (See Table 7.2.)

As with most things, moderation is best. Too little or too much dietary fat can be harmful. The National Academy of Sciences has recommended that 20 to 35% of your daily calories should come from fats.

Proteins

Proteins are complex organic compounds made up of **amino acids.** They contain approximately 4 calories per gram. They are essential for growth and repair of body tissues, including muscle. Proteins are a potential source of energy but are not normally used for fuel when carbohydrates and fats are available.

Of the 20 amino acids that make up proteins, 9 are essential in your diet because your body cannot produce them. A food that contains all essential amino acids is called a **complete protein.** Foods from animal sources such as fish, poultry, meat, eggs, and dairy products are complete proteins. **Incomplete proteins** come from plant sources such as beans, peas, grains, and nuts. By

combining some selected incomplete proteins, such as beans and rice, you can get all of the essential amino acids in adequate amounts.

Nutrient Summary

Your body needs adequate amounts of water, minerals, vitamins, carbohydrates, fats, and proteins. All of these are necessary in your daily food intake. In each case, a deficiency creates a problem, an adequate amount is optimal, and more is not better. To get the nutrients that you need, eat a variety of good foods and drink at least eight glasses of water a day.

The National Academy of Sciences has suggested the following guideline for caloric intake for adults:

- 45 to 65% from carbohydrates
- 10 to 35% from proteins
- 20 to 35% from fats
- Less than 7% from saturated fats

(See Figure 7.2.)

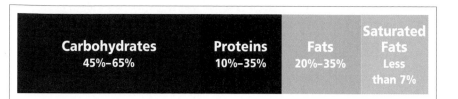

Carbohydrates 45%–65%	Proteins 10%–35%	Fats 20%–35%	Saturated Fats Less than 7%

Figure 7.2 A balanced diet.
Guidelines from The National Academy of Sciences, 2002.

The "Secret" Weight Training Diet

Many weight trainers and athletes are looking for the "secret" or "magic" diet that will make them successful and produce miraculous results. The truth is that the "secret" diet is a balanced diet that includes all the nutrients your body needs in the correct amounts, and it is different for every individual. The information in this chapter will help you develop your own individualized "secret" weight training diet that works for you.

The major difference between the diet that is best for the average sedentary adult and the diet that is best for the active athlete or weight trainer is the total number of calories consumed. Athletes and weight trainers often need to consume more calories because they burn more calories.

Fundamental principles of the "secret" weight training diet are moderation, variety, and balance. The diet should consist of a wide variety of good quality food in the proper amounts. You need to eat right to gain healthy muscle tissue and remove excess stored body fat.

Choose foods that have high **nutrient density.** These are foods that are high in nutrients compared to calories. By contrast, **junk foods** have low-nutrient density. They are foods that are high in calories and low in nutrients. Carbonated drinks and potato chips do not produce quality muscle but certainly can be stored as fat. Remove the junk food from your diet and eat high-quality foods. Learn to tell the difference. One of the top bodybuilders in the world claimed that his bodybuilding success was 80% nutrition and 20% training.

Tools for Healthy Eating

Three important tools to help you develop a healthy eating plan are food labels, the Dietary Guidelines for Americans, and MyPyramid.

Food Labels

Food labels provide important information to guide you in eating a healthy, balanced diet. The labels focus on the nutrients most clearly associated with health and disease risk. See Figure 7.3 for more information on food labels.

Dietary Guidelines for Americans

The second tool to help you develop a healthy eating plan is the Dietary Guidelines for Americans. These guidelines provide science-based advice on food and physical activity choices for health. The Dietary Guidelines describe a healthy diet as one that

- Emphasizes fruits, vegetables, whole grains, and fat-free or low-fat milk and milk products.

- Includes lean meats, poultry, fish, beans, eggs, and nuts.

- Is low in saturated fats, trans fats, cholesterol, salt (sodium), and added sugars.

See Table 7.3 for key recommendations.

MyPyramid

The third tool to help you develop a healthy eating plan is MyPyramid. MyPyramid, which replaces the Food Guide Pyramid that was introduced in 1992, is part of a food guidance system that emphasizes the need for a more individualized approach to improving diet and exercise. MyPyramid translates the principles of the Dietary Guidelines for Americans to assist you in making healthier food and physical activity choices.

The USDA food guidance system provides excellent information to help you individualize your eating plan. This website features the following:

- *MyPyramid Plan* provides a quick estimate of what and how much food that you should eat from the different food groups by entering your age, gender, and activity level.

- *MyPyramid Tracker* provides more detailed information on your diet quality and physical activity status by comparing a day's worth of foods eaten with current nutrition guidance. Relevant nutrition and physical activity messages are tailored to your

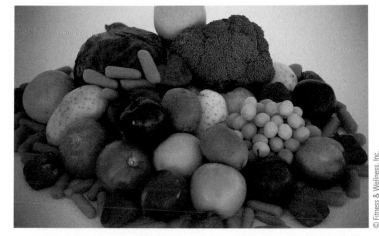

A balanced diet should include plenty of fruits and vegetables.

Key Recommendations for the General Population

Adequate Nutrients within Calorie Needs

- Consume a variety of nutrient-dense foods and beverages within and among the basic food groups while choosing foods that limit the intake of saturated and *trans* fats, cholesterol, added sugars, salt, and alcohol.
- Meet recommended intakes within energy needs by adopting a balanced eating pattern, such as the U.S. Department of Agriculture (USDA) Food Guide or the Dietary Approaches to Stop Hypertension (DASH) Eating Plan.

Weight Management

- To maintain body weight in a healthy range, balance calories from foods and beverages with calories expended.
- To prevent gradual weight gain over time, make small decreases in food and beverage calories and increase physical activity.

Physical Activity

- Engage in regular physical activity and reduce sedentary activities to promote health, psychological well-being, and a healthy body weight.
  - To reduce the risk of chronic disease in adulthood: Engage in at least 30 minutes of moderate-intensity physical activity, above usual activity, at work or home on most days of the week.
  - For most people, greater health benefits can be obtained by engaging in physical activity of more vigorous intensity or longer duration.
  - To help manage body weight and prevent gradual, unhealthy body weight gain in adulthood: Engage in approximately 60 minutes of moderate- to vigorous-intensity activity on most days of the week while not exceeding caloric intake requirements.
  - To sustain weight loss in adulthood: Participate in at least 60 to 90 minutes of daily moderate-intensity physical activity while not exceeding caloric intake requirements. Some people may need to consult with a healthcare provider before participating in this level of activity.
- Achieve physical fitness by including cardiovascular conditioning, stretching exercises for flexibility, and resistance exercises or calisthenics for muscle strength and endurance.

Food Groups to Encourage

- Consume a sufficient amount of fruits and vegetables while staying within energy needs. Two cups of fruit and 2½ cups of vegetables per day are recommended for a reference 2,000-calorie intake, with higher or lower amounts depending on the calorie level.
- Choose a variety of fruits and vegetables each day. In particular, select from all five vegetable subgroups (dark green, orange, legumes, starchy vegetables, and other vegetables) several times a week.
- Consume 3 or more ounce-equivalents of whole-grain products per day, with the rest of the recommended grains coming from enriched or whole-grain products. In general, at least half the grains should come from whole grains.
- Consume 3 cups per day of fat-free or low-fat milk or equivalent milk products.

Fats

- Consume less than 10 percent of calories from saturated fatty acids and less than 300 mg/day of cholesterol, and keep *trans* fatty acid consumption as low as possible.
- Keep total fat intake between 20 to 35 percent of calories, with most fats coming from sources of polyunsaturated and monounsaturated fatty acids, such as fish, nuts, and vegetable oils.
- When selecting and preparing meat, poultry, dry beans, and milk or milk products, make choices that are lean, low-fat, or fat-free.
- Limit intake of fats and oils high in saturated and/or *trans* fatty acids, and choose products low in such fats and oils.

Carbohydrates

- Choose fiber-rich fruits, vegetables, and whole grains often.
- Choose and prepare foods and beverages with little added sugars or caloric sweeteners, such as amounts suggested by the USDA Food Guide and the DASH Eating Plan.

- Reduce the incidence of dental caries by practicing good oral hygiene and consuming sugar- and starch-containing foods and beverages less frequently.

Sodium and Potassium

- Consume less than 2,300 mg (approximately 1 teaspoon of salt) of sodium per day.
- Choose and prepare foods with little salt. At the same time, consume potassium-rich foods, such as fruits and vegetables.

Alcoholic Beverages

- Those who choose to drink alcoholic beverages should do so sensibly and in moderation—defined as the consumption of up to one drink per day for women and up to two drinks per day for men.
- Alcoholic beverages should not be consumed by some individuals, including those who cannot restrict their alcohol intake, women of childbearing age who may become pregnant, pregnant and lactating women, children and adolescents, individuals taking medications that can interact with alcohol, and those with specific medical conditions.
- Alcoholic beverages should be avoided by individuals engaging in activities that require attention, skill, or coordination, such as driving or operating machinery.

Food Safety

- To avoid microbial foodborne illness:
  - Clean hands, food contact surfaces, and fruits and vegetables. Meat and poultry should not be washed or rinsed.
  - Separate raw, cooked, and ready-to-eat foods while shopping, preparing, or storing foods.
  - Cook foods to a safe temperature to kill microorganisms.
  - Chill (refrigerate) perishable food promptly and defrost foods properly.
  - Avoid raw (unpasteurized) milk or any products made from unpasteurized milk, raw or partially cooked eggs or foods containing raw eggs, raw or undercooked meat and poultry, unpasteurized juices, and raw sprouts.

Note: The *Dietary Guidelines for Americans 2005* contains additional recommendations for specific populations. The full document is available at www.healthierus.gov/dietaryguidelines.

Table 7.3 Dietary Guidelines for Americans 2005

1. The Serving Size

The first place to start when you look at the Nutrition Facts label is the serving size and the number of servings in the package. Serving sizes are standardized to make it easier to compare similar foods; they are provided in familiar units, such as cups or pieces, followed by the metric amount, e.g., the number of grams. **Pay attention to the serving size, especially how many servings there are in the food package.** In the sample label, one serving of macaroni and cheese equals one cup. If you ate the whole package, you would eat **two** cups.

2. Calories (and Calories from Fat)

Calories provide a measure of how much energy you get from a serving of this food. Many Americans consume more calories than they need without meeting recommended intakes for a number of nutrients. The calorie section of the label can help you manage your weight.

In the example, there are 250 calories in one serving of this macaroni and cheese. How many calories from fat are there in ONE serving? Answer: 110 calories, which means almost half the calories in a single serving come from fat.

The Nutrients: How Much?

Look at the top of the nutrient section in the sample label. It shows you some key nutrients that impact on your health and separates them into two main groups:

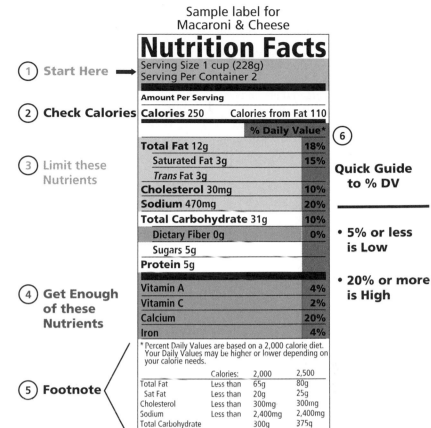

Sample label for Macaroni & Cheese

Nutrition Facts

Serving Size 1 cup (228g)
Serving Per Container 2

Amount Per Serving

Calories 250	Calories from Fat 110

	% Daily Value*
Total Fat 12g	18%
Saturated Fat 3g	15%
Trans Fat 3g	
Cholesterol 30mg	10%
Sodium 470mg	20%
Total Carbohydrate 31g	10%
Dietary Fiber 0g	0%
Sugars 5g	
Protein 5g	

Vitamin A	4%
Vitamin C	2%
Calcium	20%
Iron	4%

* Percent Daily Values are based on a 2,000 calorie diet. Your Daily Values may be higher or lower depending on your calorie needs.

	Calories:	2,000	2,500
Total Fat	Less than	65g	80g
Sat Fat	Less than	20g	25g
Cholesterol	Less than	300mg	300mg
Sodium	Less than	2,400mg	2,400mg
Total Carbohydrate		300g	375g
Dietary Fiber		25g	30g

① **Start Here** →

② **Check Calories**

③ **Limit these Nutrients**

④ **Get Enough of these Nutrients**

⑤ **Footnote**

⑥ **Quick Guide to % DV**

- 5% or less is Low
- 20% or more is High

3. Limit These Nutrients

The nutrients listed first are the ones Americans generally eat in adequate amounts, or even too much. They are identified in yellow as **Limit these Nutrients.** Eating too much fat, saturated fat, *trans* fat, cholesterol, or sodium may increase your risk of certain chronic diseases, like heart disease, some cancers, or high blood pressure.

4. Get Enough of These

Most Americans don't get enough dietary fiber, vitamin A, vitamin C, calcium, and iron in their diets. They are identified in blue as **Get Enough of these Nutrients**. Eating enough of these nutrients can improve your health and help reduce the risk of some diseases and conditions.

Remember: You can use the Nutrition Facts label not only to help *limit* those nutrients you want to cut back on but also to *increase* those nutrients you need to consume in greater amounts.

5. Understanding the Footnote on the Bottom of the Nutrition Facts Label

Note the * used after the heading "% Daily Value" on the Nutrition Facts label. It refers to the Footnote in the lower part of the nutrition label, which tells you **"%DVs are based on a 2,000 calorie diet"**. It doesn't change from product to product, because it shows recommended dietary advice for all Americans—it is not about a specific food product. DVs are recommended levels of intakes. DVs in the footnote are based on a 2,000 or 2,500 calorie diet. Note how the DVs for some nutrients change, while others (for cholesterol and sodium) remain the same for both calorie amounts.

6. The Percent Daily Value (%DV)

The % Daily Values (%DVs) are based on the Daily Value recommendations for key nutrients but only for a 2,000 calorie daily diet—not 2,500 calories. You, like most people, may not know how many calories you consume in a day. But you can still use the %DV as a frame of reference whether or not you consume more or less than 2,000 calories.

Do you need to know how to calculate percentages to use the %DV? No, the label (the %DV) does the math for you. It helps you interpret the numbers (grams and milligrams) by putting them all on the same scale for the day (0–100%DV). The %DV column doesn't add up vertically to 100%. Instead each nutrient is based on 100% of the daily requirements for that nutrient (for a 2,000 calorie diet). This way you can tell high from low and know which nutrients contribute a lot, or a little, to your **daily** recommended allowance (upper or lower). **Five %DV or less is low** for all nutrients, those you want to limit (e.g., fat, saturated fat, cholesterol, and sodium), or for those that you want to consume in greater amounts (fiber, calcium, etc). **Twenty %DV or more is high** for all nutrients.

Note that *Trans* fat, sugars, and protein do not list a %DV on the Nutrition Facts label. No daily reference value has been established. For more information on Food Labeling see *http://www.cfsan.fda.gov/label.html* Adapted from the FDA/Center for Food Safety & Applied Nutrition

Figure 7.3 Understanding food labels

desire to maintain your current weight or to lose weight.

- *Inside MyPyramid* provides in-depth information for every food group, including recommended daily amounts in commonly used measures, like cups and ounces, with examples and everyday tips. The section also includes recommendations for choosing healthy oils, discretionary calories, and physical activity.

- *Start Today* provides tips and resources that include downloadable suggestions on all the food groups and physical activity and a worksheet to track what you are eating.

Go to the MyPyramid website to access the information you need to develop a plan that is individualized for your needs and caloric requirements. For an *example* of an eating plan for a 2000-calorie diet, see Figure 7.4 (p. 48). **To develop your personal eating plan, complete the MyPyramid Worksheet found at www.mypyramid.gov.** See Figure 7.5 (p. 49) for a *sample* worksheet for a 2000-calorie diet.

Healthy Body Composition

Healthy body composition includes avoiding excessive body fat while developing and maintaining muscle tissue. The development and maintenance of healthy body composition requires a combination of weight training, aerobic exercise, and healthy eating.

Fat Loss

Concerns about fat loss are increasing for many Americans, and these concerns are justified. There is an "epidemic of obesity" in the United States. According to the National Center for Chronic Disease Prevention and Health Promotion, an estimated 61% of adults are either overweight or obese.

At any given time, 33 to 40% of women and 20 to 24% of men are trying to lose weight. Another 28% of all adults are trying to maintain a weight loss, usually without success. The simple and well-documented truth is that diet alone is not an effective weight-loss strategy. Only about 10% of the people who begin a diet without exercise are able to lose the desired weight. Only 1 in 200 can maintain the weight loss for any significant amount of time. Diets alone don't work.

So what is the key to body-fat management? The formula is to maintain a moderate level of total calories, minimize fat calories, and get regular exercise. A well-rounded exercise program including aerobic exercise, weight training, and flexibility activities is best for body-fat management and overall fitness. It is vital to incorporate both exercise and nutrition principles for successful fat loss and management.

Continuous, rhythmic activities that use large muscle groups are good for high-caloric expenditure. Examples of good fat-loss activities are walking, cycling, and jogging. Combining aerobic exercises with weight training exercises produces even better results.

How does weight training fit into a fat-loss program? When you start a weight training program, you will gain muscle and lose fat. Therefore, you may not see an immediate loss of total body weight. To lose excess body fat, you should perform longer training sessions consisting of more sets, repetitions, and exercises, which will use more total calories. You cannot "spot reduce" body fat. For example, sit-ups do not "spot reduce" fat from your abdominal area.

Weight training increases lean body mass, which includes muscle, bone, ligaments, and tendons. Because of the high-energy needs of muscle tissue, more calories are required to maintain muscle tissue than fat tissue. Each additional pound of muscle tissue can raise your basal metabolic rate by as much as 35 calories per day. Weight training increases lean body mass (muscle), which in turn increases your metabolic rate. This results in greater caloric expenditure even when you are not exercising.

Because weight training increases muscle mass (calorie-burning cells), it is also beneficial for people who are at their recommended body weight but have a higher than recommended percentage of body fat.

An added benefit of weight training is the firm and fit appearance that results from regular training. Muscle tissue is more dense than fat tissue, so increasing muscle tissue and decreasing fat tissue results in a trim, healthy, toned appearance.

The secret to healthy weight loss is found in the following guidelines:

1. Eat a balanced diet of good-quality food.

2. Do not skip meals, and eat smaller meals.

3. Do not omit any food groups but reduce portion sizes.

4. Decrease your total caloric intake by about 500 to 1000 calories per day. This should translate into a safe 1 to 2 pounds of fat loss per week.

5. Increase your level of physical activity. Develop and follow a planned exercise program.

6. Select daily activities where food is not easily available.

7. Keep moving. Stay active. Your metabolic rate and caloric expenditure are higher when you are awake and moving than when you are sleeping and resting.

8. Eat more slowly. Your brain needs about 20 minutes to register that you are full.

Eating six or seven times a day can make it easier to lose body fat by keeping you from getting extremely hungry. Extreme hunger can lead to overeating and fat storage. By eating smaller amounts more often, every 2 or 3 hours, you don't get as hungry. By spreading your food intake throughout the day, you experience a steady energy level and avoid the "food coma" that follows a big meal and the "energy slump" that occurs between big meals.

Fruits make excellent midmorning, midafternoon, and after-dinner snacks. Fruit is naturally packaged, low in calories, low in fat, high in vitamins and minerals, and often sweet in taste. Many people crave "sweets" because they don't eat enough fruit. Eating six or seven times a day allows you to plan your caloric intake better and reduce your hunger sensation.

Muscle Gain

Achieving a healthy body composition requires more than reducing excessive body fat. It also includes increasing lean body mass. Here are some tips to help you gain muscle:

- Perform brief weight training workouts.
- Work the largest muscles in your body.
- Eat a balanced diet of high-quality foods.
- Increase your total caloric intake by 500 to 1000 calories per day.
- Eat smaller meals and more frequently.
- Get plenty of rest. Slow down, stay calm, and decrease your other activities.
- Set a healthy goal to gain muscle and not just total body weight. Watch your body-fat level. Any diet in which caloric intake exceeds caloric need can lead to fat storage and unhealthy weight gain.

Eating six or seven smaller meals per day makes it easier to increase your total daily caloric intake than eating three times a day. Small meals take less time to eat and keep your body fueled all day.

So whether you are trying to lose excess body fat, gain muscle, or some combination of the two, you will experience greater success if you plan your food intake carefully. Combining healthy eating with proper exercise is the key to healthy body composition.

Supplements

Beginning weight trainers frequently ask about the value of using dietary supplements as part of their weight training program. When you are eating according to the recommendations of the USDA as outlined in the Dietary Guidelines and MyPyramid, you will be consuming a balanced diet of high-quality foods that should meet all of your nutritional needs. Independent researchers (those who do not sell food supplements) have found no benefits from the use of supplements when the subjects were on a healthy diet that was meeting all of their nutritional needs.

If you have dietary deficiencies, supplements might be beneficial, but you should improve your diet before resorting to "quick-fix" supplements to make up for your poor eating habits. If you suspect that you have dietary deficiencies, consult with a nutrition expert such as a dietitian.

The purpose of this book is to encourage a lifelong pattern of healthy weight training exercise supported by healthy eating. There are entire books on supplements. Before you decide to take a supplement, you should research it completely. Ask the following questions:

- **Does it work?** How do you know it works? Who says it works—independent researchers, those selling supplements, or someone you met in the weight room?
- **Is it necessary?** Could you get the same benefit from spending your money on high-quality food and healthy eating? Do you want to buy and take this supplement for the rest of your life?
- **Is it safe?** What scientific evidence is available to prove that the supplement is safe?
- **Is it legal?** Do you know the penalty for possession and use if it is not legal?
- **Is it a banned substance?** If you are an athlete, is this a substance that has been banned by a sports governing body like the NCAA, NFL, NBA, USOC, or IOC?

Don't take chances with your health. If you choose to use supplements, be absolutely certain that they are safe, effective, and legal.

Protein Supplementation

Most Americans do not need more protein. For adult men and women, the recommendation for protein intake is 0.8 gram per kilogram of body weight. Heavy, intense, high-volume strength training can increase this requirement to 1.7 grams of protein per kilogram of body weight.

Muscle requires the right kind and amount of exercise to stimulate growth and enough nutrients in a healthy diet to build muscle tissue. A balanced diet can provide all the protein you need.

Sports Drinks

Most people who exercise for an hour or less in moderate temperatures need only water to replace fluids. The electrolytes lost will be replaced by a balanced diet. For longer periods of exertion or exercise in hot and humid conditions, however, the American Dietetic Association suggests a sports beverage as part of the hydration-replacement process. Sports drinks replace fluid and electrolytes that are lost during exercise and provide energy to working muscles.

Rest

Although weight training exercise is the stimulus, the positive changes in the muscular system as a result of weight training take place between exercise sessions as your body rebuilds and adapts to the exercise overload. Adequate rest and nutrition are necessary for these positive changes to occur.

Weight training progress is best when a muscle receives 2 to 4 days of rest between exercise sessions. Fewer than 2 days of rest or more than 4 days of rest between workouts results in slower progress.

An average amount of sleep is 8 hours per night. Sleep requirements, however, vary from one person to another and for the same person based upon changes in activity levels. At first, beginning weight trainers may find that they need more sleep to recover from this new demand. As they become accustomed to the increased physical activity and their bodies begin to function more efficiently, they often return to normal sleep patterns.

"Hard gainers"—individuals who have a hard time gaining muscle—sometimes need as many as 10 hours of sleep each night. Some "easy gainers" gain muscle on 7 hours of sleep per night.

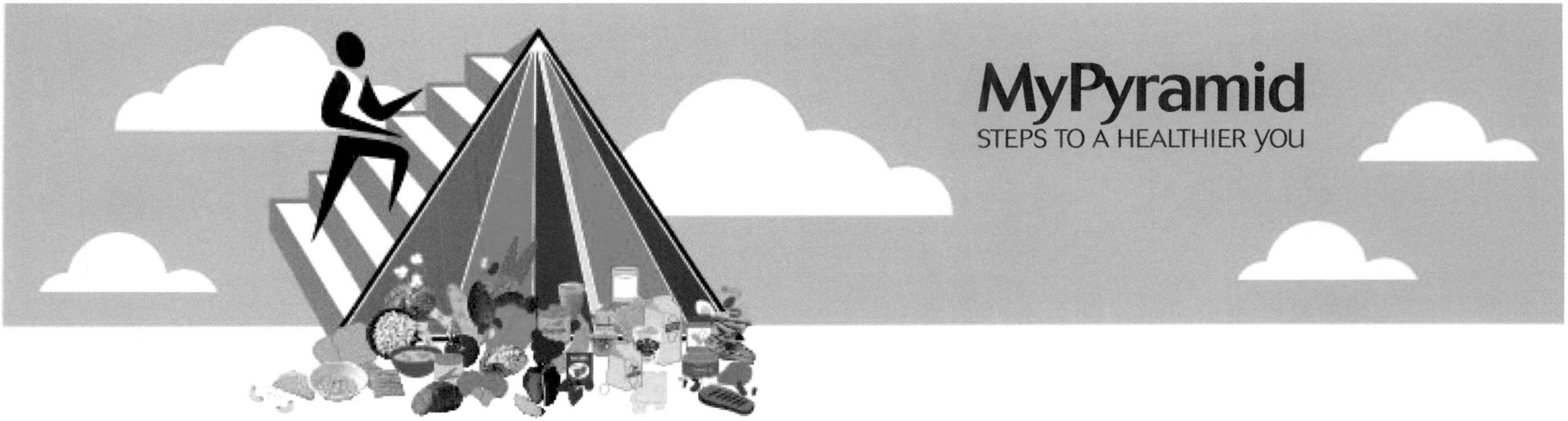

MyPyramid
STEPS TO A HEALTHIER YOU

Based on the information you provided, this is your daily recommended amount from each food group.

GRAINS
6 ounces

Make half your grains whole

Aim for at least **3 ounces** of whole grains a day

VEGETABLES
2 1/2 cups

Vary your veggies

Aim for these amounts **each week:**

Dark green veggies
= 3 cups

Orange veggies
= 2 cups

Dry beans & peas
= 3 cups

Starchy veggies
= 3 cups

Other veggies
= 6 1/2 cups

FRUITS
2 cups

Focus on fruits

Eat a variety of fruit

Go easy on fruit juices

MILK
3 cups

Get your calcium-rich foods

Go low-fat or fat-free when you choose milk, yogurt, or cheese

MEAT & BEANS
5 1/2 ounces

Go lean with protein

Choose low-fat or lean meats and poultry

Vary your protein routine—choose more fish, beans, peas, nuts, and seeds

Find your balance between food and physical activity

Be physically active for at least **30 minutes** most days of the week.

Know your limits on fats, sugars, and sodium

Your allowance for oils is **6 teaspoons** a day.

Limit extras—solid fats and sugars—to **265 calories a day.**

Name: _____

Your results are based on a pattern.

This calorie level is only an estimate of your needs. Monitor your body weight to see if you need to adjust your calorie intake.

Figure 7.4 The MyPyramid **example** of a 2000-calorie diet

Source: U.S. Department of Agriculture Center for Nutrition Policy and Promotion, April 2005.

MyPyramid Worksheet

Check how you did today and set a goal to aim for tomorrow

MyPyramid.gov
STEPS TO A HEALTHIER YOU

Write in Your Choices for Today	Food Group	Tip	Goal Based on a 2000 calorie pattern.	List each food choice in its food group*	Estimate Your Total
	GRAINS	Make at least half your grains whole grains	6 ounce equivalents (1 ounce equivalent is about 1 slice bread, 1 cup dry cereal, or 1/2 cup cooked rice, pasta, or cereal)		_____ ounce equivalents
	VEGETABLES	Try to have vegetables from several subgroups each day	2 1/2 cups Subgroups: Dark Green, Orange, Starchy, Dry Beans and Peas, Other Veggies		_____ cups
	FRUITS	Make most choices fruit, not juice	2 cups		_____ cups
	MILK	Choose fat-free or low fat most often	3 cups (1 1/2 ounces cheese = 1 cup milk)		_____ cups
	MEAT & BEANS	Choose lean meat and poultry. Vary your choices—more fish, beans, peas, nuts, and seeds	5 1/2 ounce equivalents (1 ounce equivalent is 1 ounce meat, poultry, or fish, 1 egg, 1 T. peanut butter, 1/2 ounce nuts, or 1/4 cup dry beans)	*Some foods don't fit into any group. These "extras" may be mainly fat or sugar—limit your intake of these.	_____ ounce equivalents
	PHYSICAL ACTIVITY	Build more physical activity into your daily routine at home and work.	At least 30 minutes of moderate to vigorous activity a day, 10 minutes or more at a time.		_____ minutes

How did you do today?   ☐ Great   ☐ So-So   ☐ Not so Great

My food goal for tomorrow is: _____

My activity goal for tomorrow is: _____

Figure 7.5 The MyPyramid worksheet for a **sample** 2000-calorie diet

Source: U.S. Department of Agriculture, Center for Nutrition Policy and Promotion, April 2005.

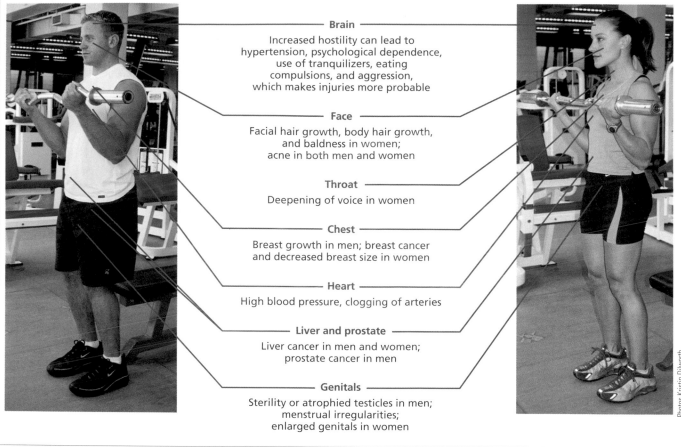

Photos Kristin Dilworth

Figure 7.6 Adverse effects of steroids on parts of the body

Not getting adequate rest can be one of the greatest obstacles to weight training progress for young adults. Many high school students, college students, and young adults train hard with weights but do not get enough sleep to recover completely from their training sessions.

Weight training is intense and demanding. Too many other physical activities will slow your weight training progress. If you want to maximize your weight training gains, you should cut down on other physically strenuous activities. Young adults (ages 16 to 30) often wear themselves out with a large number of activities. This combination of too much activity and not enough rest can cancel out all the hard work you put into your weight training exercises. Some experienced weight trainers believe that they progress better if they train hard for 6 to 8 weeks, take

1 week off, and then start a new training program.

As you get older, some of your bodily functions will naturally begin to slow down. You should not view this as a totally negative experience. Many older adults report that they need less sleep, less food, and less exercise to stay healthy and physically fit. Beyond an approximate age of 40 or 50, two weight training workouts per week might be sufficient to maintain the muscular system in excellent condition. This depends on your weight training goals and your personal ability to recover from your workouts.

Some days you will feel better than others. On some days you likely will not feel like doing your normal workout. On those days you probably should train anyway but reduce your intensity and your total workload. You should not skip workouts completely on those

days. You should maintain the frequency of workouts. Once you skip a training session, it becomes easier to skip another and another until soon you have no training schedule at all. It is easy to stop training completely and difficult to get started again. Many people begin weight training, but few have what it takes to continue for the rest of their lives. *Persistence* is a common word but a rare human quality.

The only time you should not train is when you are sick or injured. If you are truly physically sick, you should not work out because it will further stress your body. You cannot "sweat out" a cold or any other illness. Instead, you should follow your doctor's advice and rest completely so that you can get well in the shortest possible time. If you keep training, an illness can drag on for weeks, and you probably will not experience any progress despite your training efforts.

Weight training should contribute to your health. When you are not well, you should stop training, get well, and then start again. If you are sick more than two or three times a year, you should examine your lifestyle.

If you feel exhausted when you wake up and are sleepy all day long, even during activities you normally enjoy, you may not be getting enough rest. If you are sleeping about 8 hours each night but are still feeling tired, you may be overtraining. In that case, try reducing the total number of sets in your weight training program and see if you feel better. Adequate rest and recovery time are essential to your weight training progress.

Drugs

The drugs discussed here are anabolic steroids, alcohol, and tobacco. Although the topic of drugs is much broader, these are the ones that are most prominent in weight trainers.

Anabolic Steroids

One drug problem in weight training is the use of **anabolic steroids,** synthetic compounds that are like the natural hormones the body produces. Most of the steroids that weight trainers and athletes use to gain muscle mass are similar to the hormone testosterone.

Anabolic steroids are thought to promote muscle growth. They have been difficult to study because they also produce highly undesirable and dangerous side effects. Therefore, they can be studied only at safe (low) levels. Athletes who claim that steroids work take massive doses—sometimes 10 to 20 times greater than the safe dose an ethical physician would allow in a research study with human subjects.

Steroid use is dangerous because it can produce serious, life-threatening side effects and adverse reactions. (See Figure 7.6.) The side effects for women are just as dangerous as they are for men. Some of the undesirable side effects that users have reported and doctors have observed include endocrine disturbances, atrophy of the testicles, male impotency, liver damage, liver cancer, psychological disturbances, and coronary artery disease. The effects on specific parts of the body are given in Figure 7.6.

Steroid users agree that steroids work only when accompanied by extremely hard weight training. Therefore, steroids are not "easy gain" muscle drugs that replace hard work. Intense workouts are still necessary to gain muscle. This is another reason that steroid effects are hard to study. It is difficult to determine how much of the improvement is a result of training and how much can be attributed to the steroid effect.

Many steroid users have reported an increase in aggressiveness. This can result in more intense weight training workouts, which might produce greater gains. Because anabolic steroids do not produce scientifically proven and predictable benefits and they do have documented and dangerous side effects, their use is not recommended. Some young lifters and bodybuilders who are taking steroids are causing lifelong damage to their bodies that they will regret when they get older. Steroid abuse has also caused a number of deaths.

Weight training is an activity that should improve your health and natural performance level. Drug use and abuse have no place in a health development program such as *weight training for life.*

Alcohol

No evidence is available to suggest that a low level of alcohol consumption (one drink per day or less) interferes with weight training progress. Neither is any evidence available indicating that alcohol has any beneficial effect on weight training progress. But heavy alcohol consumption does have profound detrimental effects on your body (Figure 7.7). If your desire is to have a strong and healthy body, you need to keep your alcohol consumption to a minimum or eliminate it completely.

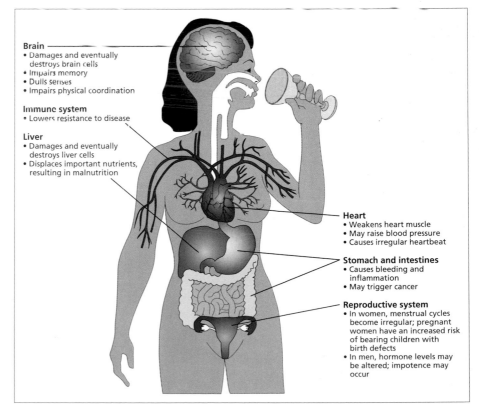

Brain
- Damages and eventually destroys brain cells
- Impairs memory
- Dulls senses
- Impairs physical coordination

Immune system
- Lowers resistance to disease

Liver
- Damages and eventually destroys liver cells
- Displaces important nutrients, resulting in malnutrition

Heart
- Weakens heart muscle
- May raise blood pressure
- Causes irregular heartbeat

Stomach and intestines
- Causes bleeding and inflammation
- May trigger cancer

Reproductive system
- In women, menstrual cycles become irregular; pregnant women have an increased risk of bearing children with birth defects
- In men, hormone levels may be altered; impotence may occur

Figure 7.7 Long-term risks associated with chronic alcohol use

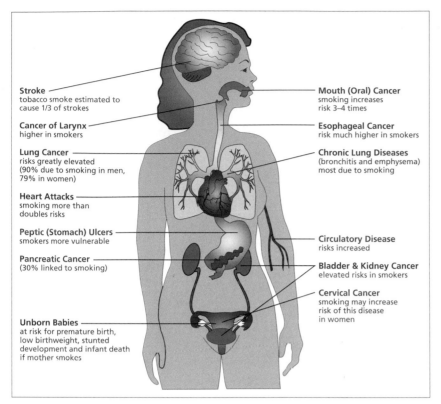

Figure 7.8 Adverse health effects of smoking

Stroke
tobacco smoke estimated to
cause 1/3 of strokes

Cancer of Larynx
higher in smokers

Lung Cancer
risks greatly elevated
(90% due to smoking in men,
79% in women)

Heart Attacks
smoking more than
doubles risks

Peptic (Stomach) Ulcers
smokers more vulnerable

Pancreatic Cancer
(30% linked to smoking)

Unborn Babies
at risk for premature birth,
low birthweight, stunted
development and infant death
if mother smokes

Mouth (Oral) Cancer
smoking increases
risk 3–4 times

Esophageal Cancer
risk much higher in smokers

Chronic Lung Diseases
(bronchitis and emphysema)
most due to smoking

Circulatory Disease
risks increased

Bladder & Kidney Cancer
elevated risks in smokers

Cervical Cancer
smoking may increase
risk of this disease
in women

Tobacco

Smoking or chewing tobacco has no known beneficial effects, but smoking does harm the respiratory and circulatory systems (Figure 7.8). It decreases performance and training capacity. Smoking reduces the ability to finish demanding weight training workouts and interferes with the ability to recover from workouts. Smoking and chewing tobacco both have been proven to cause cancer and other diseases, and neither will help you reach your weight training goals.

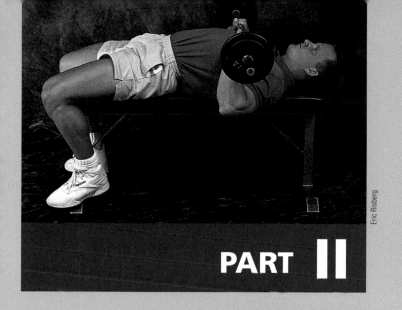

Eric Risberg

PART II

Learning More Weight Training Exercises

The weight training exercises in this book are arranged into the following chapters:

Chapter 8: Chest Exercises
Chapter 9: Back Exercises
Chapter 10: Shoulder Exercises
Chapter 11: Arm Exercises
Chapter 12: Leg Exercises
Chapter 13: Trunk Flexion and Extension Exercises

The exercise descriptions in this book are consistent with the exercise technique recommendations of the National Strength and Conditioning Association (NSCA). The general pattern in these chapters is to present a basic barbell and dumbbell exercise on the left page along with a description of the

exercise and an illustration of the major muscles used to perform the exercise. Then, on the right page directly across from it are common exercise machine positions for the same exercise.

Various exercise machines have been used here because of the many good ones on the market. The idea is for you to recognize that you can either perform the basic barbell or dumbbell exercise or perform the same exercise movement on the machines that you have available and realize that you are working the same muscles.

Some exercise machines use a cam or a pivot system to vary the resistance as you move through the range of motion. This is not really important for you to understand as a beginner as long as you provide your muscles with an appropriate overload stimulus.

The **concentric phase** of a weight training exercise is the portion of the exercise during which your muscular contractions overcome the resistance and the weight is lifted. The **eccentric phase** of a weight training exercise is the portion of the exercise during which the resistance overcomes your muscular contraction and the weight is lowered. The same muscles are working during both the concentric phase and the eccentric phase of a weight training exercise.

Almost any barbell exercise can also be performed using dumbbells. In many dumbbell exercises, the dumbbells may be moved together or in an alternating manner.

Major Muscles of the Human Body

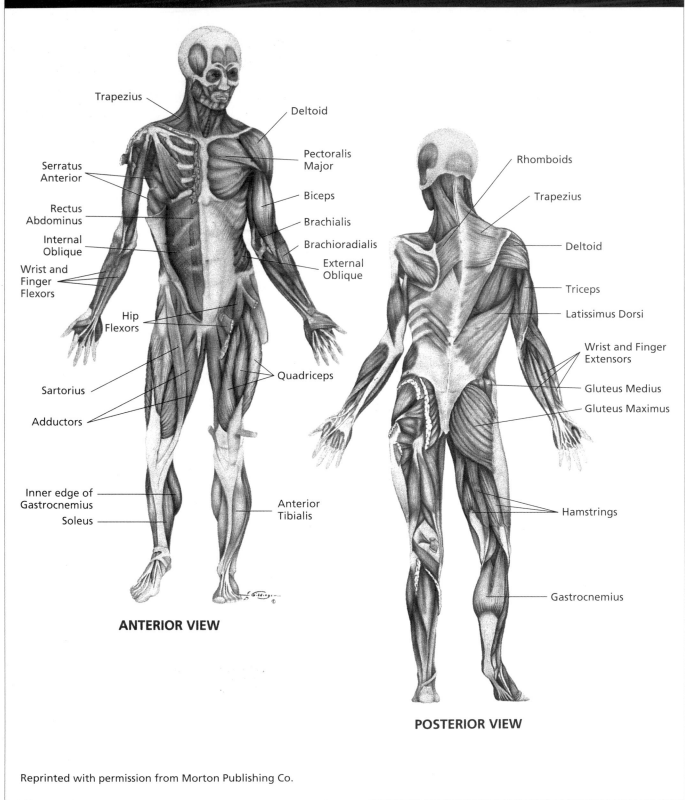

ANTERIOR VIEW

POSTERIOR VIEW

Reprinted with permission from Morton Publishing Co.

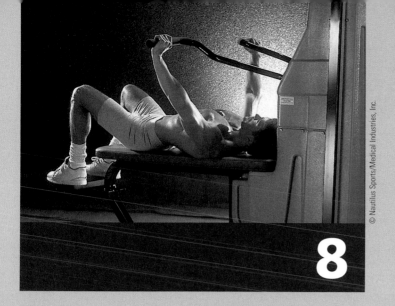

© Nautilus Sports/Medical Industries, Inc.

8

Chest Exercises

Chest (Pectoralis Major)

Barbell Bench Press
Dumbbell Bench Press
Prone Bench Press Machine
Seated Chest Press Machine

Incline Barbell Bench Press
Incline Dumbbell Bench Press
Incline Bench Press Machine
Incline Bench Press Machine

Dumbbell Bent-Arm Flyes
Machine Bent-Arm Flyes
Pec Deck Machine
Chest Machine

Chest/Back (Pectoralis Major and Latissimus Dorsi)

Barbell Bent-Arm Pullover
Dumbbell Straight-Arm Pullover
Bent-Arm Pullover Machine
Pullover Machine

CHEST (PECTORALIS MAJOR)

Bench Press

___**Muscles developed:** Pectoralis major, anterior deltoid, triceps.

___**Starting position:** Start on your back on a flat bench; hold a barbell directly above your shoulders, arms straight, and both feet flat on the floor (A).

___**Eccentric phase:** Inhale as you lower the bar to touch your chest (B).

___**Concentric phase:** Exhale as you press the weight back up to the starting position.

___**Spotting:** Have a spotter stand at the head end of the bench in case you cannot press the weight back to the starting position.

___**Variations:** Change the angle of the bench and change the width of the hand spacing on the bar to achieve many variations of this basic chest exercise. You also may choose to perform this exercise with dumbbells.

___**Additional information:** To make this exercise easier, use a rack to hold the weight above the bench. Some people prefer to place their feet on the bench to keep the lower back flat on the bench.

___**Caution:** Do not arch your lower back during this lift. Use a spotter.

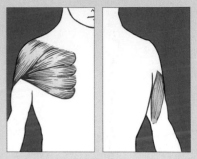

Front   Back

Barbell

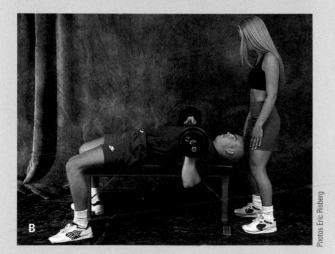

Dumbbell

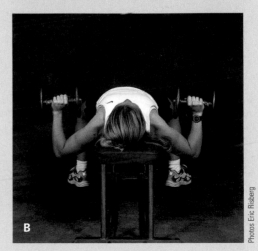

Photos Eric Risberg

Prone Bench Press Machine

___**Muscles developed:** Pectoralis major, anterior deltoid, triceps.

___**Starting position:** Start on your back on a flat bench; grasp the bar with your hands wider than shoulder-width and your elbows bent; place both feet flat on the floor or on the end of the bench (A).

___**Concentric phase:** Exhale as you press the weight upward to a straight-arm position (B).

___**Eccentric phase:** Inhale as you lower the weight to the starting position.

___**Cautions:**

1. Do not arch your lower back or lift your hips off the bench when you do this lift.

2. Keep your head a safe distance away from the weight stack and the selector pin.

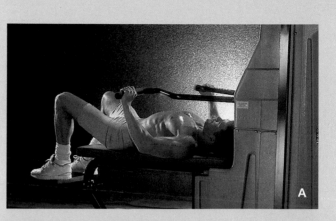

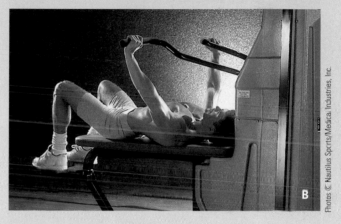

Photos © Nautilus Sports/Medical Industries, Inc.

Seated Chest Press Machine

___**Muscles developed:** Pectoralis major, anterior deltoid, triceps.

___**Starting position:** Adjust the machine so that you start in a seated position with the exercise handles at chest level. Grasp the exercise handles with your hands wider than shoulder-width and your elbows bent (A).

___**Concentric phase:** Exhale as you press forward to a straight arm position (B).

___**Eccentric phase:** Inhale as you allow the weight to return to the starting position.

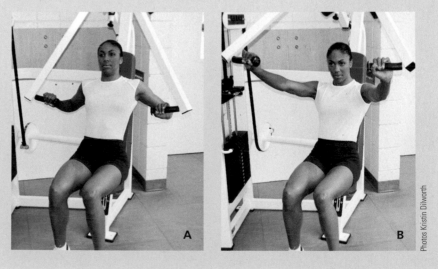

Photos Kristin Dilworth

Incline Bench Press

___ **Muscles developed:** Upper pectoralis major, anterior deltoid, triceps.

___ **Starting position:** Start on your back on an incline bench; hold a barbell directly above your shoulders with both arms straight and both feet flat on the floor (A).

___ **Eccentric phase:** Inhale as you lower the bar to touch your chest (B).

___ **Concentric phase:** Exhale as you press the weight back up to the starting position.

___ **Spotting:** Have a spotter stand behind the bench in case you cannot get the weight back to the starting position.

___ **Variations:**

1. Change the angle of the incline bench.

2. Change your hand spacing on the bar.

3. Use dumbbells instead of a barbell.

___ **Additional information:** To make this exercise easier to perform, use a weight rack to support the weight above the bench.

___ **Caution:** Dumbbells can be difficult to control because they are free to move in any direction. Begin with a light weight and master the movement before using heavier dumbbells. Have a spotter in position to help if you begin to lose control of the exercise movement.

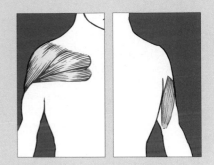

Front   Back

Barbell

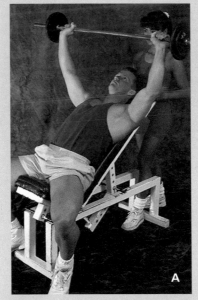

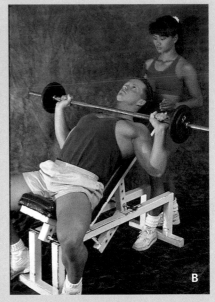

A

B

Photos Eric Risberg

Dumbbell

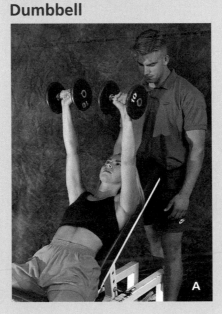

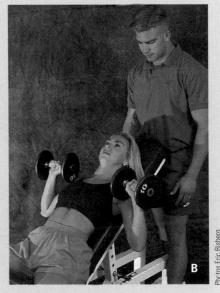

A

B

Photos Eric Risberg

Incline Bench Press Machine

___**Muscles developed:** Upper pectoralis major, anterior deltoid, triceps.

___**Starting position:** Start in a seated position on an incline bench press machine (A).

___**Concentric phase:** Exhale as you press the weight upward to a straight arm position (B).

___**Eccentric phase:** Inhale as you slowly lower the weight to the starting position.

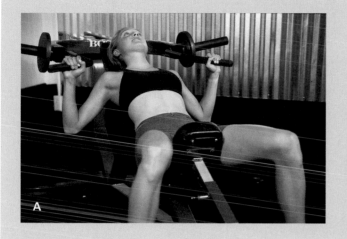
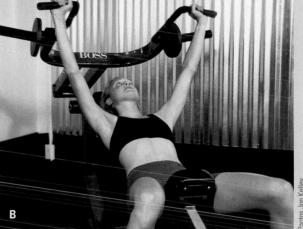

Photos Jon Kelley

Incline Bench Press Machine

___**Muscles developed:** Upper pectoralis major, anterior deltoid, triceps.

___**Starting position:** Start in a seated position on an incline bench press machine (A).

___**Concentric phase:** Exhale as you press the weight upward to a straight arm position (B).

___**Eccentric phase:** Inhale as you slowly lower the weight to the starting position.

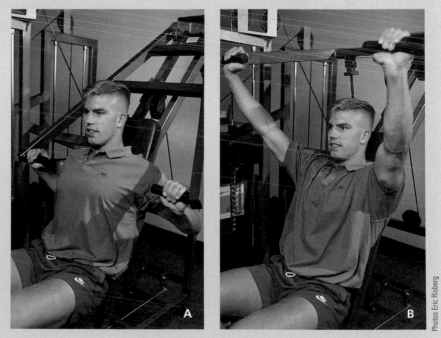

Photos Eric Risberg

Bent-Arm Flyes

___ **Muscles developed:** Pectoralis major, anterior deltoid.

___ **Starting position:** Start on your back on a flat exercise bench; hold one dumbbell in each hand above your shoulders, with your arms slightly bent (A).

___ **Eccentric phase:** Inhale as you move the dumbbells away from each other and lower them toward the floor (B).

___ **Concentric phase:** Exhale as you return the dumbbells to the starting position.

___ **Variations:** Perform this exercise on an incline or decline bench.

___ **Caution:** Keep your elbows slightly bent throughout this exercise to place the exercise stress on the pectoralis major muscle and relieve the stress on the elbow joint.

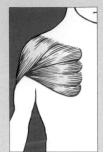

Front

Dumbbell

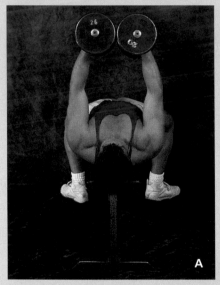

A

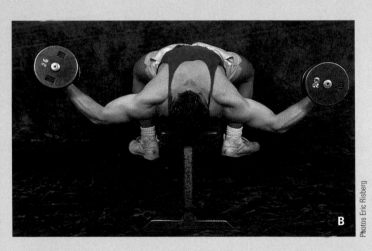

B

Photos Eric Risberg

Machine Flyes

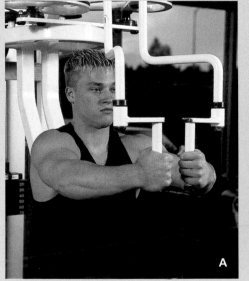

A

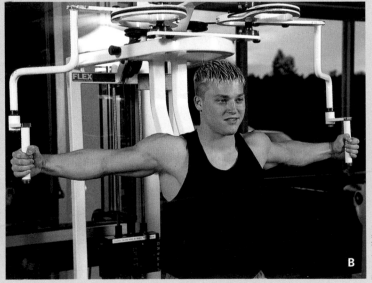

B

Photos Jon Kelley

Pec Deck Machine

___**Muscles developed**: Pectoralis major, anterior deltoid.

___**Starting position:** Start in a seated position with your elbows bent and your forearms on the padded exercise bars. Adjust the seat so that your elbows are shoulder height (A).

___**Concentric phase:** Exhale as you pull your arms forward and toward each other. Keep pulling until the exercise bars gently touch each other (B).

___**Eccentric phase:** Inhale as you slowly allow your arms to return to the starting position.

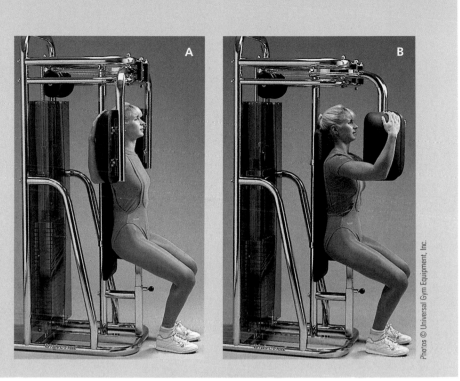

Photos © Universal Gym Equipment, Inc.

Chest Machine

___**Muscles developed:** Pectoralis major, anterior deltoid.

___**Starting position:** Start on your back on the bench and place your arms under the padded exercise bars. (See photo.)

___**Concentric phase:** Exhale as you pull your bent arms upward and toward each other. Keep pulling until the exercise bars gently touch each other or come to the end of their travel. Pause briefly and try to squeeze your arms together.

___**Eccentric phase:** Inhale as you slowly allow your arms to return to the starting position.

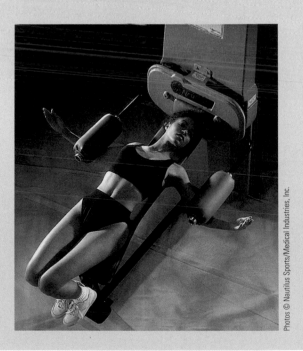

Photos © Nautilus Sports/Medical Industries, Inc.

CHEST / BACK
(PECTORALIS MAJOR AND LATISSIMUS DORSI)

Barbell Bent-Arm Pullover

___ **Muscles developed:** Latissimus dorsi, pectoralis major.

___ **Starting position:** Start on your back on a flat bench; hold a barbell supported on your chest, hands 6–12 inches apart, elbows bent, and head beyond the end of the bench (A).

___ **Eccentric phase:** Inhale as you lower the weight past your face toward the floor (B).

___ **Concentric phase:** Exhale as you pull the weight back to the starting position.

___ **Additional information:** Keep your elbows bent and your arms in close to your head.

___ **Caution:** Keep your arms pressed inward toward each other to avoid placing too much strain on the medial side or inside of your elbow joints.

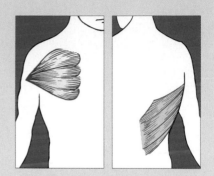

Front   Back

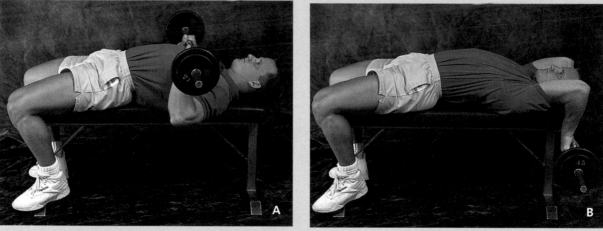

Dumbbell Straight-Arm Pullover

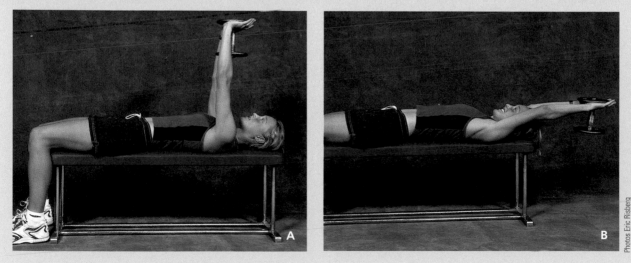

Bent-Arm Pullover Machine

___**Muscles developed:** Pectoralis major, latissimus dorsi.

___**Starting position:** Start in a seated position with your shoulder joints aligned with the pivot point of the machine. Fasten the seat belt to hold your hips in the correct position. Grasp the exercise bar behind your head with a palms-up grip (A).

___**Concentric phase:** Exhale as you pull the exercise bar over your head and all the way to your abdomen (B).

___**Eccentric phase:** Inhale as you slowly allow the bar to return to the starting position.

___**Caution:** Push on the elbow pads more than pull with your hands.

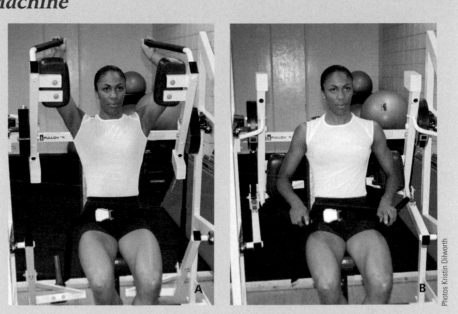

Photos Kristin Dilworth

Pullover Machine

___**Muscles developed:** Pectoralis major, latissimus dorsi.

___**Starting position:** Start in a seated position with your shoulder joints aligned with the pivot point of the pullover machine. Fasten the seat belt to hold your hips in the correct position. Push down on the foot bar to bring the exercise bar forward to a position where you can place your upper arms on the padded portion of the exercise bar as shown in the photograph (A). Allow the bar to gently pull your arms back to the starting position, then remove your feet from the foot bar.

___**Concentric phase:** Exhale as you pull the exercise bar over your head and all the way to your abdomen (B).

___**Eccentric phase:** Inhale as you slowly allow the exercise bar to return to the starting position.

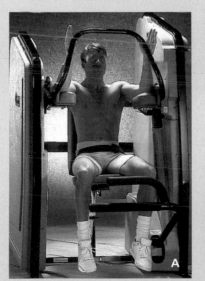
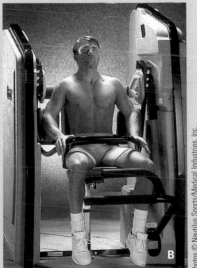

Photos © Nautilus Sports/Medical Industries, Inc.

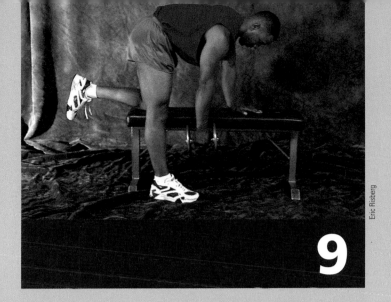

Eric Risberg

9

Back Exercises

BACK (LATISSIMUS DORSI)

Rowing

___**Muscles developed:** Latissimus dorsi, teres major, posterior deltoid, trapezius, rhomboids.

___**Starting position:** Bend over with your knees slightly bent; hold a barbell in your hands with your arms straight so that the barbell is hanging directly below your shoulders (A).

___**Concentric phase:** Exhale as the weight is pulled upward (B) until the bar touches your chest. Pause briefly with the bar held against your chest.

___**Eccentric phase:** Inhale as the weight is lowered slowly to the starting position.

___**Variations:**

1. Stand on a bench or block to get more stretch in the starting position when larger plates are used.

2. Change the distance between your hands.

3. Pull the bar to your shoulders or chest or abdomen.

4. Perform this exercise with dumbbells, bringing both up at the same time or alternately.

___**Caution:** Your lower back will be in a potentially dangerous position. To reduce the risk of injury to your lower back, keep your back flat, do not jerk or drop the weight, and keep your knees bent.

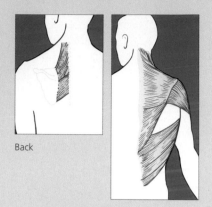

Back

Back

Barbell

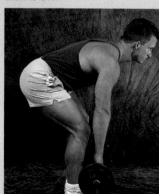

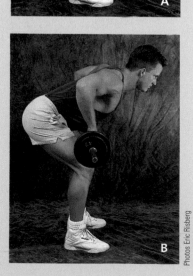

Photos Eric Risberg

One-Dumbbell

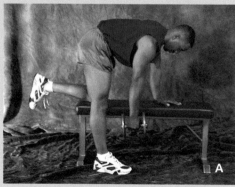

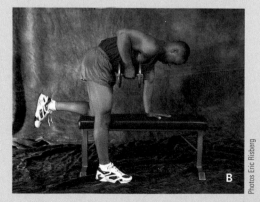

Photos Eric Risberg

Seated Rowing Machine

___**Muscles developed:** Latissimus dorsi, teres major, posterior deltoid, trapezius, rhomboids.

___**Starting position:** Adjust the chest pad so you can just reach the handles of the exercise bar with your arms fully extended (A).

___**Concentric phase:** Exhale as you pull the exercise handles toward your chest (B). Pause briefly in the fully contracted position.

___**Eccentric phase:** Inhale as you slowly allow the exercise handles to return to the starting position.

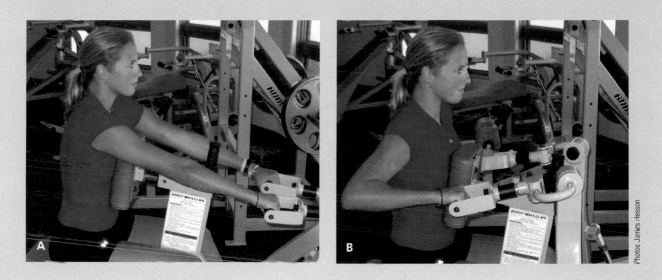

Photos James Hesson

Seated Rowing Machine

___**Muscles developed:** Latissimus dorsi, teres major, posterior deltoid, trapezius, rhomboids.

___**Starting position:** Start facing the machine and grasp one exercise bar in each hand.

___**Concentric phase:** Exhale as you pull the exercise bars toward your chest. Pause briefly in the fully contracted position and squeeze your shoulder blades together.

___**Eccentric phase:** Inhale as you slowly allow the exercise bars to return to the starting position.

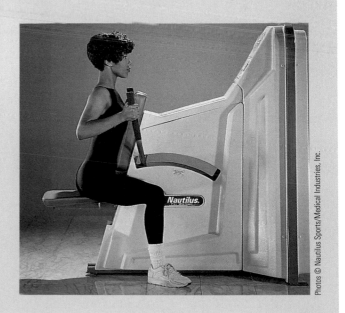

Photos © Nautilus Sports/Medical Industries, Inc.

Pull-Ups

___**Muscles developed:** Latissimus dorsi, teres major, biceps brachii.

___**Starting position:** Hang from a bar with a pronated grip (thumbs in) (A). For chin-ups use a supinated grip (thumbs out) (A).

___**Concentric phase:** Exhale as you pull yourself upward to a position with your chin above the bar (B).

___**Eccentric phase:** Inhale as you lower yourself slowly to the starting position.

___**Variations:** Change grip direction and hand spacing for variations of this exercise.

___**Additional information:** Start each pull-up from a full hang. Pause with your chin above the bar, then lower yourself slowly to the starting position. Add weight by suspending a dumbbell from a wide strap that passes around your lower back and placing the dumbbell between your thighs.

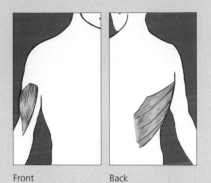

Front   Back

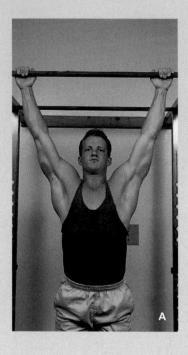

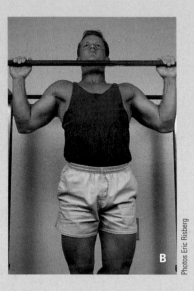

Chin-Ups

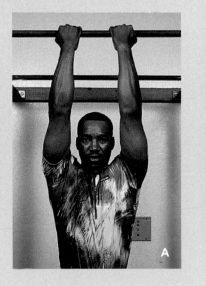

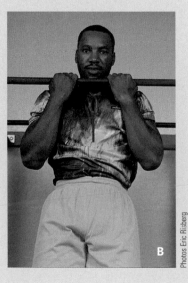

Lat Pull-Down Machine

___**Muscles developed:** Latissimus dorsi, teres major, biceps.

___**Starting position:** Grasp the bar with a pronated grip and your hands wider than shoulder width. Assume a seated position with your arms straight (A).

___ **Concentric phase:** Exhale and pull the exercise bar down to your upper chest (B). Pause briefly in the fully contracted position and squeeze your shoulder blades together.

___**Eccentric phase:** Inhale as you slowly allow the exercise bar to return to the starting position.

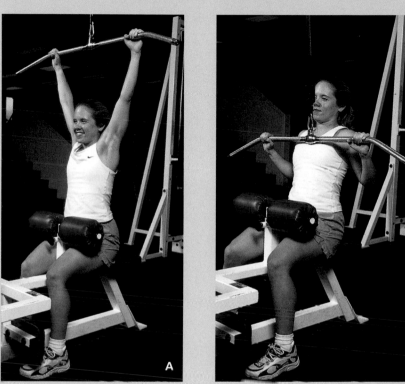

Photos Jon Kelley

Weight-Assisted Pull-Up Machine

___**Muscles developed:** Latissimus dorsi, teres major, biceps.

___**Starting position:** Set the weight for the amount of assistance you want from the machine. Grasp the overhead bar with a pronated grip. Step from the platform onto the weight-assist bar and lower yourself to the fully stretched starting position (A).

___**Concentric phase:** Exhale as you pull yourself upward to a position with your chin above the bar (B). Pause briefly and squeeze your shoulder blades together.

___**Eccentric phase:** Inhale as you lower yourself slowly to the starting position.

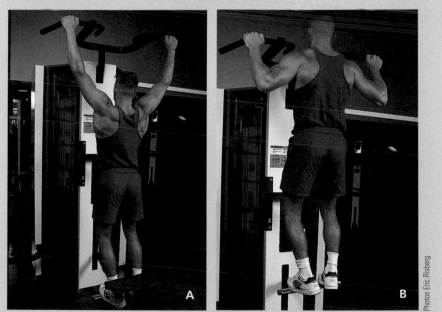

Photos Eric Risberg

UPPER BACK (TRAPEZIUS)

Shoulder Shrug

___ **Muscles developed:** Trapezius, levator scapulae.

___ **Starting position:** Start with a barbell hanging at arms length in front of your body; hold the bar with both hands in a pronated (thumbs in) grip (A).

___ **Concentric phase:** Inhale as you lift or shrug your shoulders to the highest possible position (B). Hold that position briefly.

___ **Eccentric phase:** Exhale as you slowly lower the bar to the starting position.

___ **Variations:**

1. Roll your shoulders forward and up, then back and down.

2. Roll your shoulders back and up, then forward and down.

___ **Additional information:** Do not bend your elbows or pull with your arm muscles. The hands and arms serve as hooks to hang the weight on during this exercise.

___ **Caution:** Do not jerk the weight upward or let it drop back to the starting position.

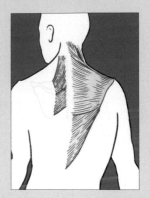

Back

Barbell

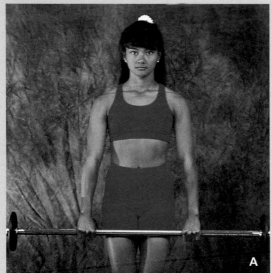

A

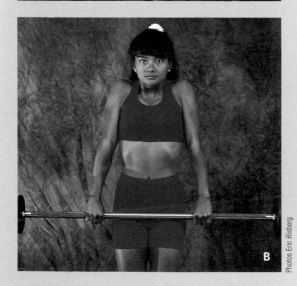

B

Photos Eric Risberg

Dumbbell

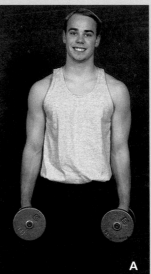

A

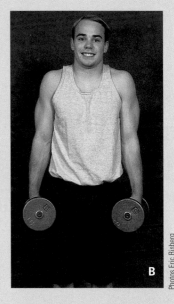

B

Photos Eric Risberg

Low Pulley Shoulder Shrug

___**Muscles developed:** Trapezius, levator scapulae.

___**Starting position:** Start in a standing position holding the low pulley handle with a pronated grip. With your arms straight, allow the weight to pull your shoulders down as far as possible (A).

___**Concentric phase:** Inhale as you pull your shoulders upward as high as possible while keeping your arms straight (B). Pause briefly and hold this position.

___**Eccentric phase:** Exhale as you slowly lower the weight to the starting position.

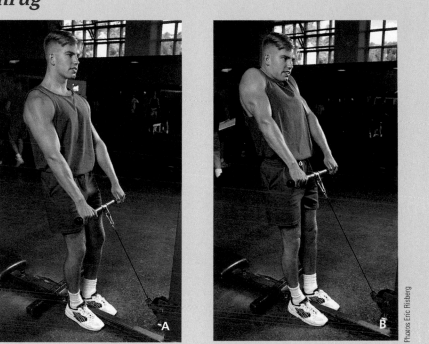

Photos Eric Risberg

Shoulder Shrug Machine

___**Muscles developed:** Trapezius, levator scapulae.

___**Starting position:** Start in a seated position with your forearms between the padded exercise bars.

___**Concentric phase:** Inhale as you pull your shoulders upward as high as possible. Pause briefly at the top of the pull and hold this position.

___**Eccentric phase:** Exhale as you slowly lower the weight to the starting position.

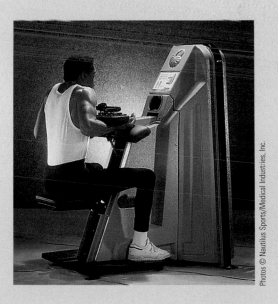

Photos © Nautilus Sports/Medical Industries, Inc.

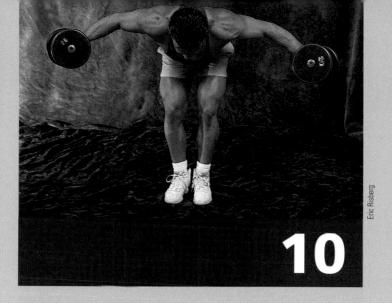
Eric Risberg

10

Shoulder Exercises

Breathing for Shoulder Exercises

When performing shoulder exercises, especially overhead lifts, there are at least three popular options for breathing:

1. *Inhale during the upward phase* and *exhale during the downward phase* of the exercise. This breathing action lifts your chest up as your arms move up and pulls your chest down as your arms move down.

2. *Exhale during the upward phase* and *inhale on the downward phase* of the exercise. This breathing action allows you to exhale during the greatest exertion of the exercise, which is the upward phase. However, it is difficult for some people to get their arms straight overhead while pulling the chest down as they exhale.

3. *Inhale deeply and lift your chest to start the upward movement phase* of the exercise and then *exhale to finish the upward phase* of the exercise.

Try all of these and see what you prefer. Find what feels natural and normal for you. There are **two cautions** that go with these breathing options.

1. Don't hold your breath and strain to lift a heavy weight.

2. Be prepared for people who have very strong opinions about which of these breathing patterns is "correct."

Shoulder (Deltoid)

Barbell Overhead Press
Dumbbell Overhead Press
Overhead Press Machine
Overhead Press Machine

Barbell Upright Rowing
Dumbbell Upright Rowing
Low Pulley Upright Rowing: Curved Bar
Low Pulley Upright Rowing: Straight Bar

Dumbbell Lateral Raise
Seated Lateral Raise Machine:
    Facing Away from Machine
Seated Lateral Raise Machine:
    Facing toward Machine

Dumbbell Front Raise
Dumbbell Bent-Over Lateral Raise

SHOULDER (DELTOID)

Overhead Press

___**Muscles developed**: Deltoid, triceps.

___**Starting position:** Start with a barbell supported at shoulder level in front of your body with your hands placed slightly wider apart than shoulder width (A).

___**Concentric phase:** Press the weight overhead to a straight-arm position (B).

___**Eccentric phase:** Slowly lower the weight to the starting position.

___**Variations:** This overhead press has many variations. The exercise can be done standing or sitting, with a barbell from the shoulders in front of the head or behind the neck, with dumbbells together, or alternating.

___**Caution:** Do not lean back or arch your back. Do not close your eyes.

___**Additional information:** This exercise is also called the military press because you stay in an erect posture (military posture) while forcing the muscles of the arms and shoulders to do all the work. Do not bend or sway the back to complete a repetition.

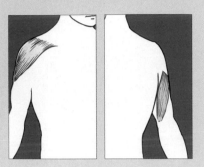

Front   Back

Barbell

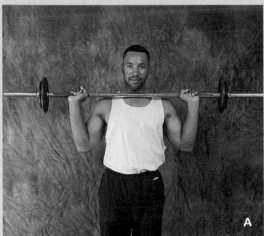

A

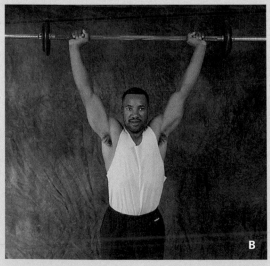

B

Photos Eric Risberg

Dumbbell

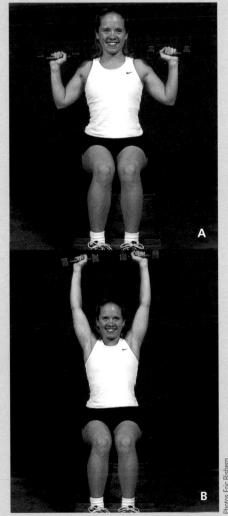

A

B

Photos Eric Risberg

Overhead Press Machine

___ **Muscles developed:** Deltoid, triceps.

___ **Starting position:** Start in a seated position. Grasp the exercise bars with your hands wider than shoulder width (A).

___ **Concentric phase:** Press the exercise bar upward to a straight-arm position (B).

___ **Eccentric phase:** Slowly lower the weight to the starting position.

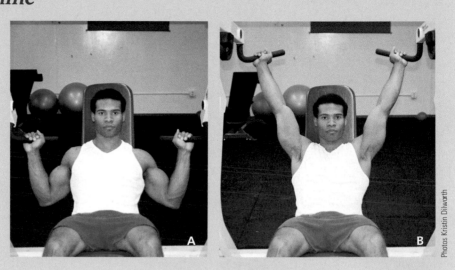

Photos Kristin Dilworth

Overhead Press Machine

___ **Muscles developed:** Deltoid, triceps.

___ **Starting position:** Start in a seated position with your back against the bench. Adjust the machine so the exercise bar handles are at shoulder height. Grasp the handles with an overgrip (thumbs in) and with your hands wider than your shoulders (A).

___ **Concentric phase:** Press the bar upward to a straight-arm position (B).

___ **Eccentric phase:** Lower the weight slowly to the starting position.

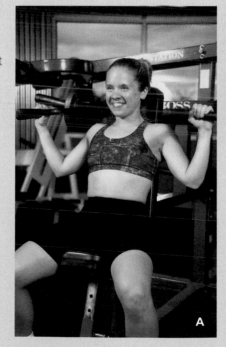
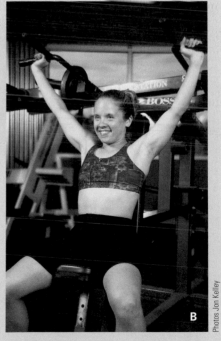

Photos Jon Kelley

Upright Rowing

___**Muscles developed:** Deltoid, trapezius.

___**Starting position:** Start with a barbell hanging at arm's length in front of your body, hands in a pronated (thumbs in) grip (A).

___**Concentric phase:** Pull your elbows upward in a smooth, continuous movement. The bar should reach shoulder level (B).

___**Eccentric phase:** Lower the bar slowly to the starting position.

___**Caution:** Concentrate on your deltoid muscles while raising your upper arm and keeping your elbows high. Your arm muscles should be as inactive as possible.

___**Additional information:** Upright rowing is like performing lateral raises.

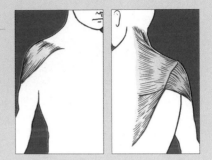

Front   Back

Barbell

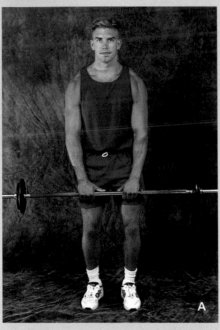

A

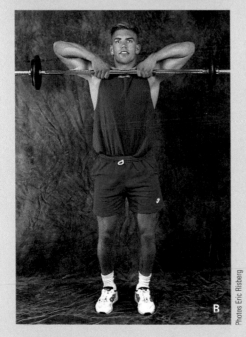

B

Photos Eric Risberg

Dumbbell

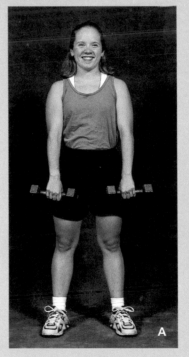

A

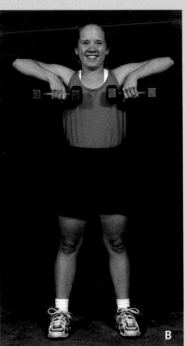

B

Photos Jon Kelley

Low Pulley Upright Rowing

___ **Muscles developed:** Deltoid, trapezius.

___ **Starting position:** Start in a standing position facing the low pulley station. Hold the exercise handle or handles on the end of the cable (A).

___ **Concentric phase:** Pull your elbows upward in a smooth, continuous movement until your hands reach shoulder height (B).

___ **Eccentric phase:** Lower the weight slowly to the starting position.

___ **Caution:** Always keep your elbows higher than your hands during this exercise.

Curved Bar

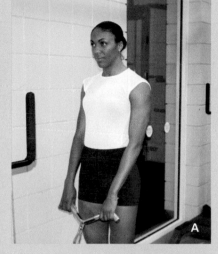
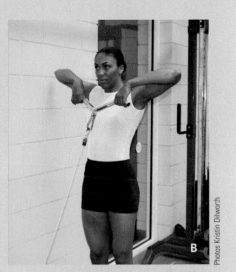

Photos Kristin Dilworth

Straight Bar

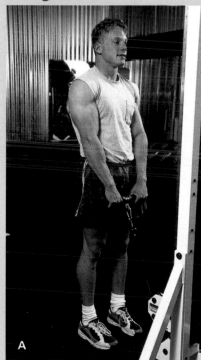
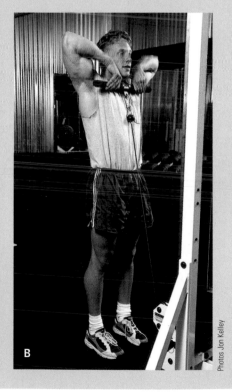

Photos Jon Kelley

Dumbbell Lateral Raise

___**Muscles developed:** Deltoid, trapezius.

___**Starting position:** Start with one dumbbell in each hand (A).

___**Concentric phase:** Lift the weights away from your body and upward. Keep your arms fairly straight and raise the weights to shoulder level (B).

___**Eccentric phase:** Lower the weights to the starting position.

___**Variations:** Perform the same exercise movement from a sitting position. The deltoid is a muscle with three fairly distinct parts: anterior (front), lateral (middle), and posterior (rear). The lateral raise tends to best develop the lateral part; the front raise develops the front part; and the bent-over lateral raise develops the rear part.

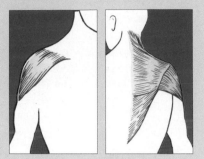

Front   Back

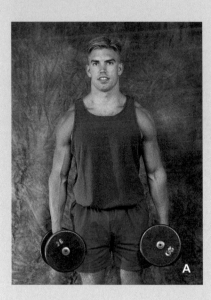

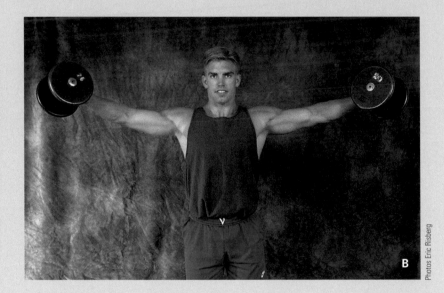

Photos Eric Risberg

Seated Lateral Raise Machine

___ **Muscles developed:** Deltoid, trapezius.

___ **Starting position:** Start in a seated position. Adjust the machine so that your shoulders are lined up with the pivot points of the machine. Place your arms against the padded portion of the exercise bars (A).

___ **Concentric phase:** Press your upper arms outward and upward to a position in which your elbows are shoulder height (B). Pause briefly at the top.

___ **Eccentric phase:** Slowly allow your arms to return to the starting position.

___ **Additional information:** To focus more on the lateral part of the deltoid, keep your forearms pointing forward.

Facing Away from Machine

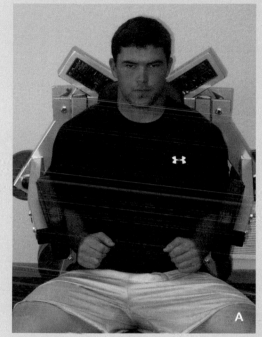

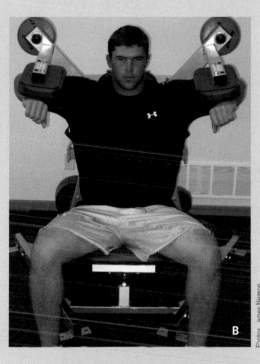

Photos James Hesson

Facing toward Machine

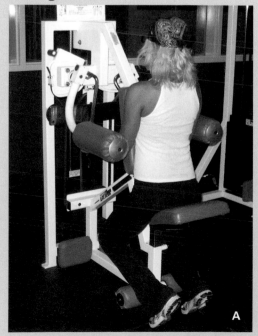

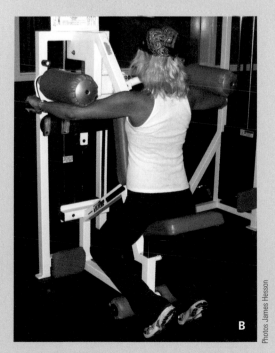

Photos James Hesson

Dumbbell Front Raise

___ **Muscles developed:** Frontal deltoid, clavicular portion of pectoralis major, coracobrachialis.

___ **Starting position:** Stand and hold a barbell or two dumbbells at arms length (A).

___ **Concentric phase:** Lift the weight to shoulder level, keeping your arms straight (B). Pause briefly.

___ **Eccentric phase:** Lower the weight to the starting position.

___ **Variations:** Raise the weight to an overhead position, as long as you do not allow your back to arch or bend.

___ **Caution:** On straight-arm exercises, a slight bend at the elbow may relieve unnecessary tension or strain in the elbow joint. This is not a problem as long as it makes the exercise more productive for you, but do not bend your elbows to make the exercise easier for the working muscles.

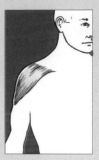

Front

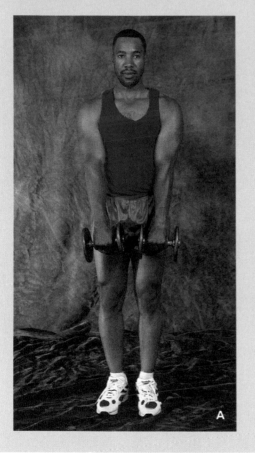

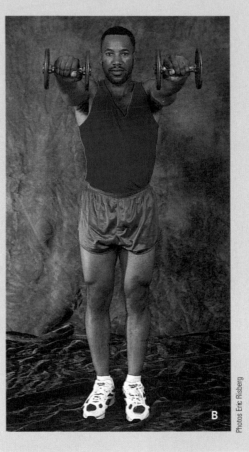

Photos Eric Risberg

Dumbbell Bent-Over Lateral Raise

___**Muscles developed:** Posterior (rear) deltoid, rhomboids, trapezius.

___**Starting position:** Bend over with your back flat and knees slightly bent; hold one dumbbell in each hand, arms straight, and dumbbells hanging directly below your shoulder joints (A).

___**Concentric phase:** Raise the dumbbells to the side up to shoulder level (B). Pause briefly.

___**Eccentric phase:** Lower the weights slowly to the starting position.

___**Variations:** Sit on the end of a bench or lie face down on a flat or incline bench that is high enough to allow your arms to hang fully extended.

___**Caution:** Lift your arms straight to the side or move them slightly forward toward your head as you lift the weight. These muscles also are developed when performing any of the rowing exercises for the back (lats).

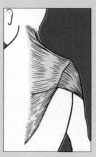

Back

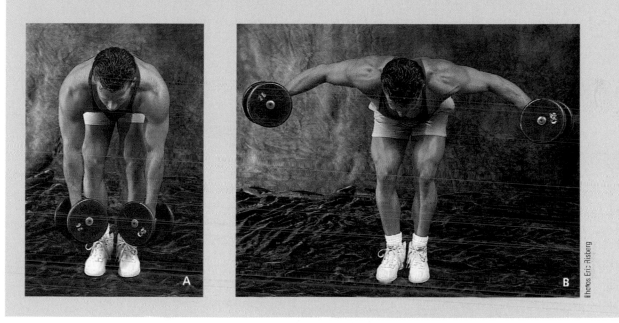

Photos Eric Risberg

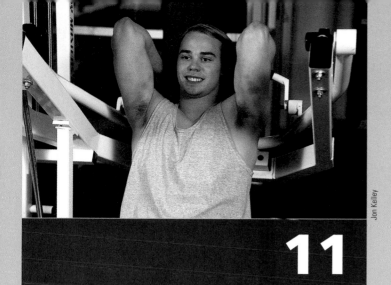

Jon Kelley

11

Arm Exercises

Upper Arm (Elbow Flexion, Biceps)

Barbell Curl
Seated Dumbbell Curl
Arm Curl Machine
Arm Curl Machine

Barbell Reverse Curl
Incline Dumbbell Curl
Preacher Curl
Low Pulley Curl

Upper Arm (Elbow Extension, Triceps)

Barbell Triceps Extension
One-Dumbbell Triceps Extension
Triceps Extension Machine
Triceps Pushdown

Parallel Bar Dips
Bench Dips
Dip Machine
Weight-Assisted Dips

Lying Triceps Extension
Close-Grip Bench Press
Triceps Extension Machine
Triceps Extension Machine

Forearm (Wrist Flexors and Wrist Extensors)

Barbell Wrist Curl
Dumbbell Wrist Curl
Reverse Barbell Wrist Curl
Reverse Dumbbell Wrist Curl

UPPER ARM (ELBOW FLEXION, BICEPS)

Barbell Curl

___**Muscles developed:** Biceps brachii, brachialis, brachioradialis.

___**Starting position:** Stand, holding a barbell in front of your body, hands gripping the bar at shoulder width with a supinated (thumbs out) grip (A).

___**Concentric phase:** Exhale while raising the weight to your shoulders by moving only at the elbow joint (B).

___**Eccentric phase:** Inhale while lowering the weight to the starting position.

___**Variations:** Any elbow flexion or curling exercise will develop the elbow flexor muscles. Curling exercises have many variations. Vary this standing curl by changing the space between your hands when gripping the bar.

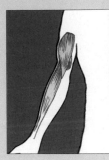

Front

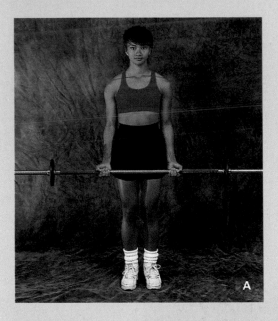

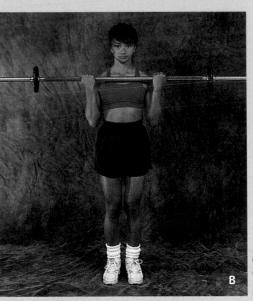

Seated Dumbbell Curl

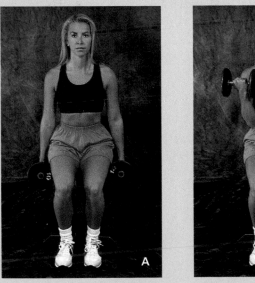

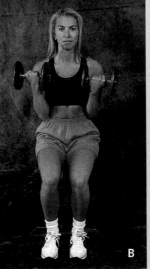

Arm Curl Machine

___**Muscles developed:** Biceps, brachialis, brachioradialis.

___**Starting position:** Grasp the exercise handles of the machine with a palms-up grip; place your elbows on the pad and line them up with the pivot point of the machine (A).

___**Concentric phase:** Exhale as you pull your hands toward your shoulders (B). When you reach the end of your elbow joint range of motion, pause briefly and hold.

___**Eccentric phase:** Inhale as you lower the weight slowly and allow your arms to return to the starting position.

___**Caution:** Do not jerk the weight up or allow it to drop and hyperextend your elbow joints at the bottom. Lift and lower the weight in a smooth, controlled manner.

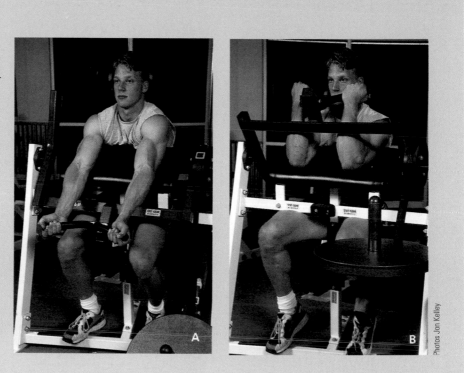

Photos Jon Kelley

Arm Curl Machine

___**Muscles developed:** Biceps, brachialis, brachioradialis.

___**Starting position:** Grasp the exercise handles of the machine with a palms-up grip; place your elbows on the pad, and line them up with the pivot point of the machine (A).

___**Concentric phase:** Exhale as you pull your hands toward your shoulders (B). When you reach the end of your elbow joint range of motion, pause briefly and hold.

___**Eccentric phase:** Inhale as you lower the weight slowly and allow your arms to return to the starting position.

___**Caution:** Do not jerk the weight up or allow it to drop and hyperextend your elbow joints at the bottom. Lift and lower the weight in a smooth, controlled manner.

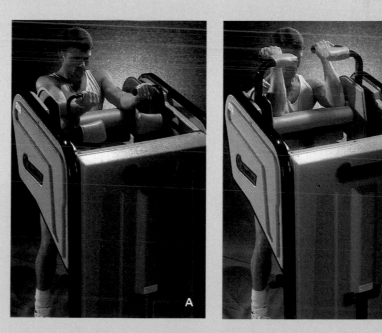

Photos © Nautilus Sports/Medical Industries, Inc.

Barbell Reverse Curl

___ **Muscles developed:** Biceps, brachialis, brachioradialis, wrist extensors, and finger flexors.

___ **Starting position:** Stand and hold a barbell in front of your body with both hands in a pronated (thumbs in) grip (A).

___ **Concentric phase:** Exhale while raising the bar to the shoulders by bending only at the elbows (B).

___ **Eccentric phase:** Inhale while lowering the bar to the starting position.

___ **Variations:** Change the distance between your hands.

___ **Additional information:** This exercise provides a strong stimulus to the forearm muscles and often is used as a forearm exercise as well as a variation of the curl.

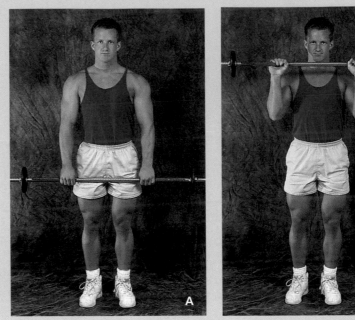

Photos Eric Risberg

Incline Dumbbell Curl

___ **Muscles developed:** Biceps brachii, brachialis, brachioradialis.

___ **Starting position:** With your back against an incline bench, hold one dumbbell in each hand with your arms extended and hanging directly below your shoulder joints (A).

___ **Concentric phase:** Exhale while bending your arms only at the elbow. Pull the weights to your shoulders (B).

___ **Eccentric phase:** Inhale while lowering weights to the starting position.

___ **Variations:**

1. Alternate your arms so that one is coming up as the other is going down.

2. Turn your arms out so the dumbbells are raised and lowered to the sides of your body instead of in front of your body.

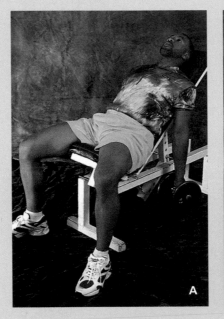
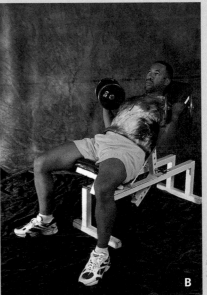

Photos Eric Risberg

Preacher Curl

___**Muscles developed:** Biceps, brachialis, brachioradialis.

___**Starting position:** Grasp the barbell or dumbbells; place your elbows on the pad and straighten your arms (A).

___**Concentric phase:** Exhale as you pull your hands toward your shoulders (B). When you reach the end of your elbow joint range of motion, pause briefly.

___**Eccentric phase:** Inhale as you lower the weight slowly and allow your arms to return to the starting position.

___**Caution:** Do not jerk the weight up. Do not allow the weight to drop and hyperextend your elbow joints at the bottom. Lift and lower the weight in a smooth, controlled manner.

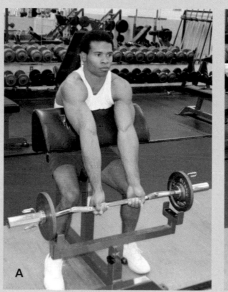
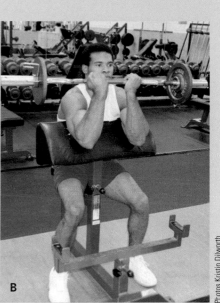

A   B

Photos Kristin Dilworth

Low Pulley Curl

___**Muscles developed:** Biceps brachii, brachialis, brachioradialis.

___**Starting position:** Stand in front of the low pulley, facing the weight stack. Hold the exercise bar in a supinated (thumbs out) grip, with both arms straight (A).

___**Concentric phase:** Exhale as you bend only at the elbow joint to bring the exercise bar up toward your shoulders. Move only your forearms; do not allow your upper arms to change position (B).

___**Eccentric phase:** Inhale as you slowly lower the bar to the starting position.

___**Variations:**

1. Change your grip spacing on the bar.

2. Use a pronated (thumbs in) grip and perform reverse curls.

___**Caution:** Bending any joint except the elbow joint will reduce the effectiveness of the exercise and increase the risk of injury.

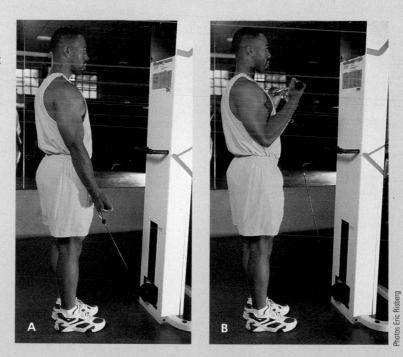

A   B

Photos Eric Risberg

UPPER ARM (ELBOW EXTENSION, TRICEPS)

Triceps Extension

___**Muscles developed:** Triceps.

___**Starting position:** Stand and hold a barbell or dumbbell overhead with both hands (A).

___**Eccentric phase:** Inhale as you slowly lower the weight behind your head (B).

___**Concentric phase:** Exhale as you extend both arms and push the weight back to the starting position.

___**Variations:**

1. Perform this exercise with a dumbbell.

2. Perform this exercise from a sitting position.

___**Additional information:** Keep your elbows up throughout the exercise.

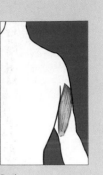

Back

Barbell

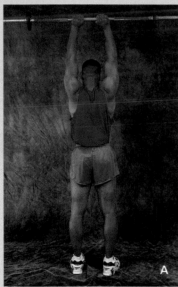

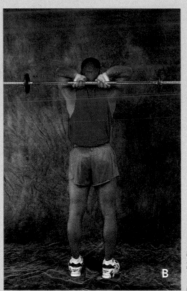

A   B

Photos Eric Risberg

One-Dumbbell

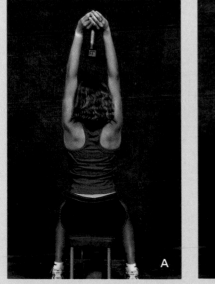

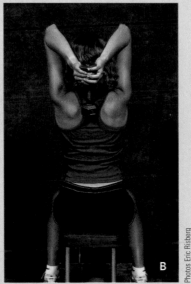

A   B

Photos Eric Risberg

Triceps Extension Machine

___ **Muscles developed:** Triceps.

___ **Starting position:** Place the little finger side of your hands or fists against the padded portion of the exercise bars. With your elbows bent, place the back of your upper arms on the pad provided and line up your elbow joints with the pivot point of the machine (A).

___ **Concentric phase:** Exhale as you push both hands forward and downward until your arms are extended. Pause briefly and hold.

___ **Eccentric phase:** Inhale as you allow your arms to slowly return to the starting position.

___ **Variations:** This exercise also may be performed one arm at a time or alternating arms (B).

___ **Caution:** Do not allow the weight to drop during the eccentric phase of the lift. Control the speed of the movement at all times.

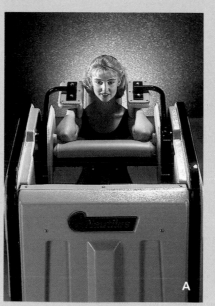
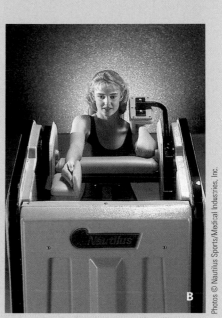

Photos © Nautilus Sports/Medical Industries, Inc.

Triceps Pushdown

___ **Muscles developed:** Triceps.

___ **Starting position:** Place both hands on the high-pulley bar (lat machine) with your palms down and your thumbs in (A).

___ **Concentric phase:** Exhale as you push the bar down until your arms are straight (B). Throughout the exercise movement, keep your upper arms by your sides and move only your hands and forearms.

___ **Eccentric phase:** Inhale as you allow your hands and forearms to slowly return to the starting position.

___ **Caution:** Keep your head, neck, and chest away from the moving cable.

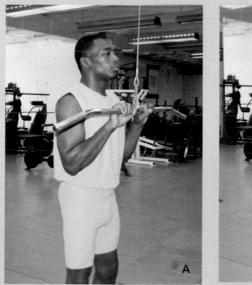
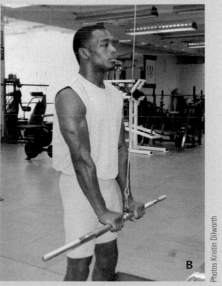

Photos Kristin Dilworth

Parallel Bar Dips

___**Muscles developed:** Triceps, pectoralis major, anterior deltoid.

___**Starting position:** Take a straight-arm support position on two bars parallel to each other and about shoulder width apart (A).

___**Eccentric phase:** Inhale as you bend your elbows and slowly lower yourself as far as possible (B).

___**Concentric phase:** Exhale as you straighten your arms and return to the starting position.

___**Additional information:** To add weight to this exercise, hang a weight or a dumbbell from a wide strap around your waist and place it between your thighs to stabilize it during the exercise.

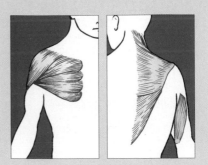

Front   Back

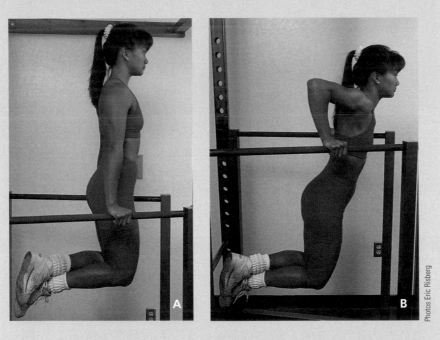

A   B

Photos Eric Risberg

Bench Dips

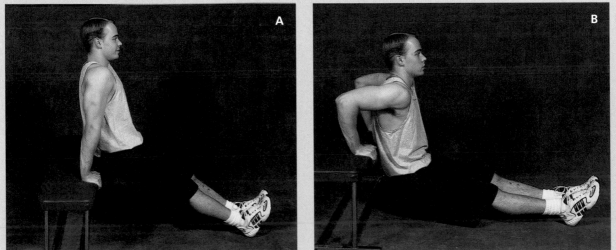

A   B

Photos Jon Kelley

Dip Machine

___**Muscles developed:** Triceps, pectoralis major, anterior deltoid.

___**Starting position:** Start with your hands on the exercise bars (A).

___**Concentric phase:** Exhale as you press the exercise bar down until your arms are straight (B).

___**Eccentric phase:** Inhale as you slowly bend your arms and allow the weight to return to the starting position.

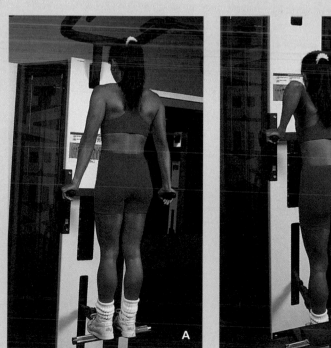

Photos Jon Kelley

Weight-Assisted Dips

___**Muscles developed:** Triceps, pectoralis major, anterior deltoid.

___**Starting position:** Select the amount of weight assistance you want from the machine. Place your hands on the parallel bars, step from the platform onto the weight assist bar, and straighten your arms (A).

___**Eccentric phase:** Inhale as you bend your elbows and slowly lower yourself as far as possible (B).

___**Concentric phase:** Exhale as you straighten your arms and return to the starting position.

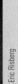

Photos Eric Risberg

Lying Triceps Extension

___**Muscles developed:** Triceps.

___**Starting positions:** Start on your back on a flat exercise bench and hold dumbbells above your shoulders, with both arms straight and your hands 6–8 inches apart (A).

___**Eccentric phase:** Inhale while lowering the dumbbells to the top of your head by bending only at your elbows (B).

___**Concentric phase:** Exhale as you push the dumbbells back to the starting position.

___**Variations:** Perform this exercise on an incline bench or a decline bench. Use one or two dumbbells or a barbell.

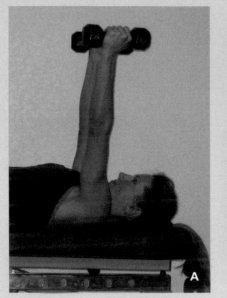

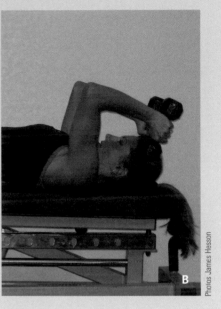

Photos James Hesson

Close-Grip Bench Press

___**Muscles developed:** Triceps, anterior deltoid, pectoralis major.

___**Starting position:** Start on your back on a flat bench and hold a barbell directly above your shoulders, with your arms straight and a close grip (hands 6–8 inches apart) (A).

___**Eccentric phase:** Inhale as you lower the bar until it touches your chest (B).

___**Concentric phase:** Exhale as you press the weight back to the starting position.

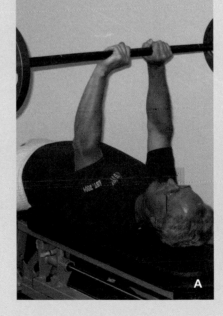

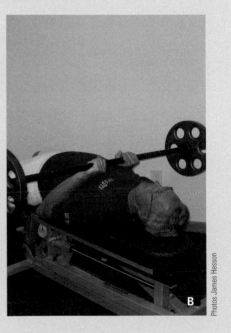

Photos James Hesson

Triceps Extension Machine

___ **Muscles developed:** Triceps.

___ **Starting position:** Sit on the triceps extension machine and grasp the bar with both elbows pointing up.

___ **Eccentric phase:** Inhale as you slowly lower the bar behind your head to the starting position.

___ **Concentric phase:** Exhale as you extend both arms and push the bar upward to a straight arm position.

___ **Caution:** Keep your elbows pointing up throughout the exercise.

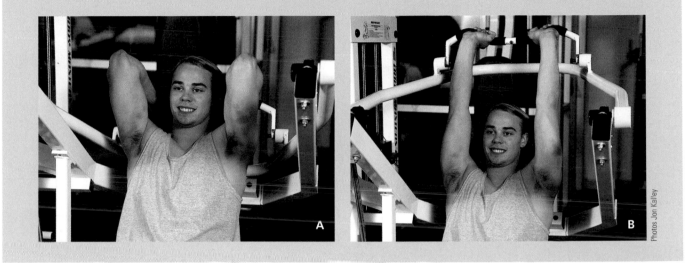

Photos Jon Kalley

Triceps Extension Machine

___ **Muscles developed.** Triceps.

___ **Starting position:** Grasp the handles of the exercise machine with your palms facing each other. With your elbows bent, place the back of your upper arms on the pad provided and line up your elbow joints with the pivot point of the machine (A).

___ **Concentric phase:** Exhale as you push both hands forward and downward until your arms are extended. Pause briefly and hold (B).

___ **Eccentric phase:** Inhale as you allow your arms to slowly return to the starting position.

___ **Caution:** Do not allow the weight to drop back to the starting position. Control the speed of movement at all times.

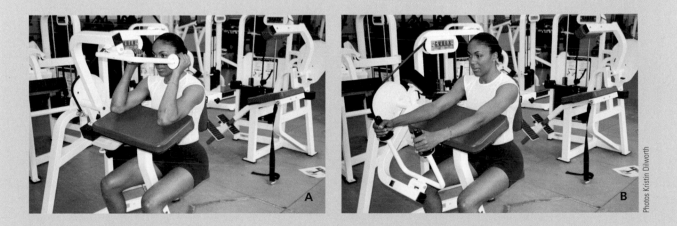

Photos Kristin Dilworth

FOREARM (WRIST FLEXORS AND WRIST EXTENSORS)

Wrist Curl

___ **Muscles developed:** Wrist and hand flexors.

___ **Starting positions:** Sit on an exercise bench and place your forearms on the bench with your wrists just beyond the end of the bench; hold a barbell with a supinated (thumbs out) grip and allow the bar to hang toward the floor (A).

___ **Concentric phase:** Lift the weight, moving only your hands and wrists (B).

___ **Eccentric phase:** Lower the bar slowly to the starting position.

___ **Variations:**

1. Use one dumbbell in each hand.

2. Use one dumbbell and exercise one arm at a time.

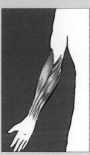

Front

Barbell

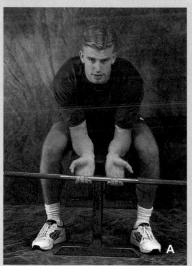
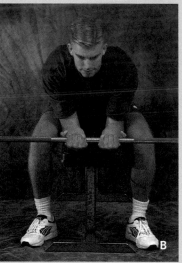

Photos Eric Risberg

Dumbbell

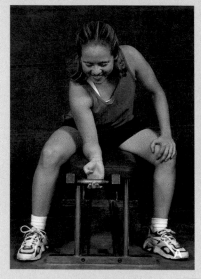
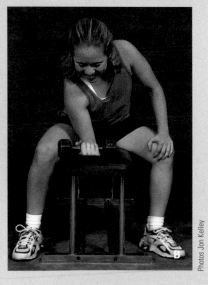

Photos Jon Kelley

Reverse Wrist Curl

___**Muscles developed:** Wrist extensors.

___**Starting position:** Sit on an exercise bench, forearms resting on top of your thighs, wrists just beyond your knees; hold a barbell, using a pronated (thumbs in) grip (A).

___**Concentric phase:** Lift the bar as high as possible, moving only at the wrist joint (B).

___**Eccentric phase:** Slowly lower the bar to the starting position.

___**Variations:**

1. Place forearms across an exercise bench.

2. Use dumbbells.

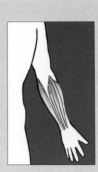

Back

Barbell

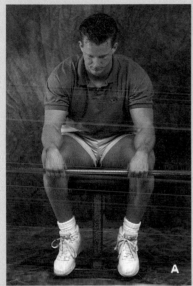

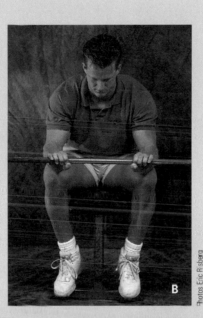

Photos Eric Risberg

Dumbbell

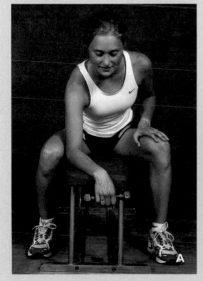

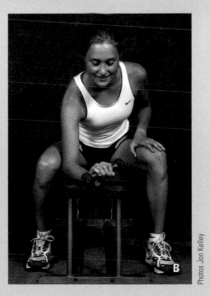

Photos Jon Kelley

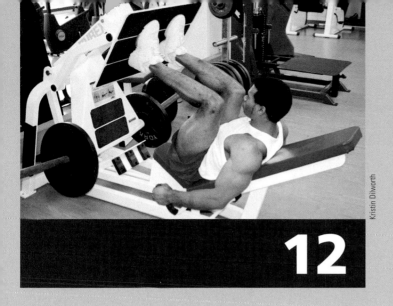
Kristin Dilworth

12

Leg Exercises

Hip and Knee Extension (Gluteus Maximus, Quadriceps, Hamstrings)

Barbell Squat
Dumbbell Squat or Dead Lift
Barbell Squat in Power Rack
Dead Lift

Squat Machine
Leg Press Machine
Leg Press Machine
Leg Press Machine

Lunge
Step Up
Leg Press Machine
Hack Squat Machine

Hip Extension (Gluteus Maximus)

Hip Extension Machine

Hip Flexion (Iliopsoas)

Hip Flexion Machine

Knee Extension (Quadriceps)

Knee Extension Machine
Knee Extension Machine

Knee Flexion (Hamstrings)

Seated Leg Curl Machine
Lying Leg Curl Machine

Ankle Plantar Flexion (Gastrocnemius, Soleus)

Standing Barbell Heel Raise
Standing Dumbbell Heel Raise
Heel Raise Machine
Standing Heel Raise Machine

One-Dumbbell Heel Raise
Heel Raise on Leg Press Machine
Heel Raise on Leg Press Machine
Seated Heel Raise

HIP AND KNEE EXTENSION
(GLUTEUS MAXIMUS, QUADRICEPS, HAMSTRINGS)

Squat

___**Muscles developed:** Quadriceps, gluteus maximus, hamstrings, erector spinae.

___**Starting position:** Stand, holding a barbell across your shoulders and upper back (A).

___**Eccentric phase:** Inhale as you bend your knees and hips while keeping your head up and your back flat. Continue bending your knees and hips until your thighs are parallel to the floor (B).

___**Concentric phase:** Exhale as you straighten your legs and hips to return to a standing position.

___**Spotting:** Have one spotter stand directly behind you or have one spotter stand at each end of the bar and one spotter stand directly behind you.

___**Caution:** Perform this exercise in a squat rack or power rack to guarantee that you will not get stuck under a heavy weight.

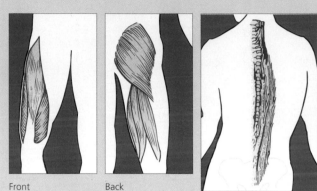

Front   Back

Back

Barbell

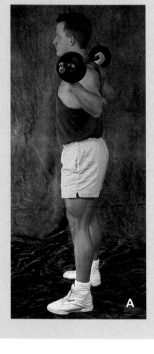

A   B

Photos Eric Risberg

Dumbbell Squat or Dead Lift

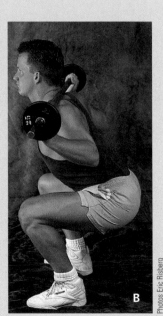
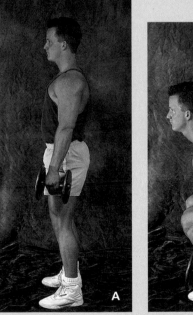

A   B

Photos Eric Risberg

Barbell Squat in Power Rack

A

B

Photos Jon Kelley

Dead Lift

___ **Muscles developed:** Erector spinae, gluteus maximus, quadriceps, hamstrings, trapezius, rhomboids, finger flexors.

___ **Starting position:** Bend over and assume a mixed grip on a barbell that is lying on the floor. Bend your knees and hips so your hips are approximately knee-level or parallel to the floor. Hold your head up and your back straight (A).

___ **Concentric phase:** Keep your neck and back straight while you pull up on the bar (B). Lift the weight by extending your hips and knees.

___ **Eccentric phase:** Keep your neck and back straight as you slowly lower the weight back to the floor by bending your knees and hips.

___ **Caution:** The dead lift is basically a hand-held squat. It is vital to maintain correct body position and progress slowly to avoid injury. When performed correctly, this is an excellent exercise to strengthen your back extensor muscles as well as your hip and knee extensors.

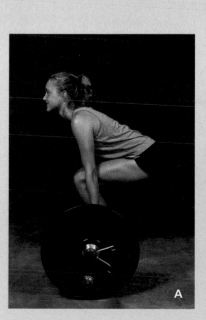

A

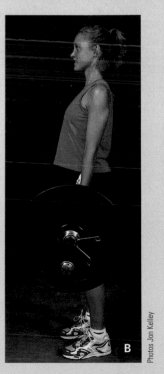

B

Photos Jon Kelley

Squat Machine

___ **Muscles developed:** Quadriceps, gluteus maximus, hamstrings, erector spinae.

___ **Starting position:** Place your shoulders under the pads and your hands on the handles. Keep your head up and your back straight. Start with your hips and knees bent (A).

___ **Concentric phase:** Exhale as you extend your knees and hips while keeping your back straight (B).

___ **Eccentric phase:** Inhale as you lower the weight slowly to the starting position by bending your knees and hips.

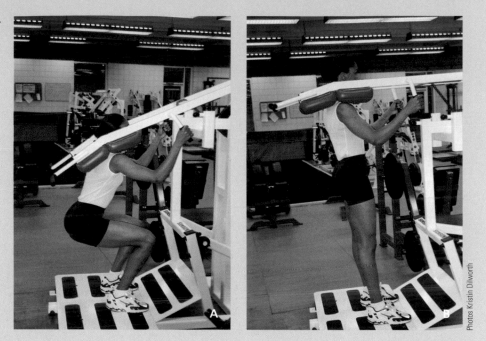

Photos Kristin Dilworth

Leg Press Machine

___ **Muscles developed:** Quadriceps, gluteus maximus, hamstrings.

___ **Starting position:** Start on your back with your shoulders against the pads, your feet on the platform shoulder width apart, and your knees bent at a 90° angle (A).

___ **Concentric phase:** Exhale as you extend your knees and hips (B).

___ **Eccentric phase:** Inhale as you bend your knees and hips and slowly return to the starting position.

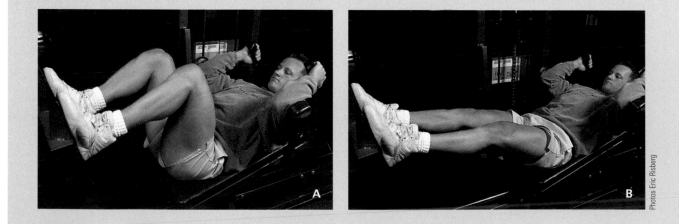

Photos Eric Risberg

Leg Press Machine

___**Muscles developed:** Quadriceps, gluteus maximus, hamstrings.

___**Starting position:** Start in a sitting position with your knees bent at a 90° angle (A).

___**Concentric phase:** Exhale as you extend your legs (B).

___**Eccentric phase:** Inhale as you bend your legs slowly and allow the weight to return to the starting position.

___**Additional information:** This exercise provides back support and therefore takes the strain off the spinal column, but it will not strengthen the back extensor muscles as the barbell squat and dead lift do.

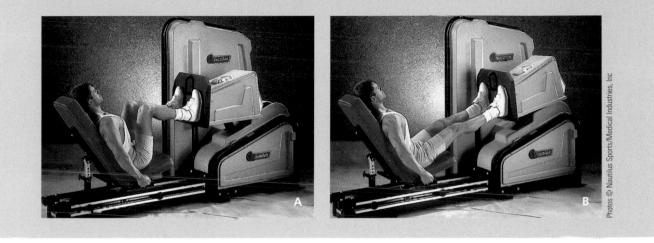

Photos © Nautilus Sports/Medical Industries, Inc

Leg Press Machine

___**Muscles developed:** Quadriceps, gluteus maximus, hamstrings.

___**Starting position:** Start in a position with your knees bent at a 90° angle (A).

___**Concentric phase:** Exhale as you extend your legs (B).

___**Eccentric phase:** Inhale as you slowly bend your legs and allow the weight to return to the starting position.

___**Additional information:** This exercise provides back support and therefore takes the strain off of the spinal column, but it will not strengthen the back extensor muscles as the barbell squat and dead lift do.

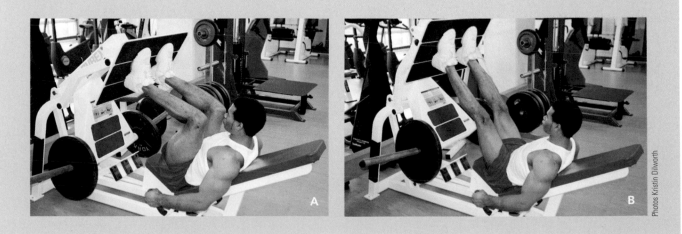

Photos Kristin Dilworth

Lunge

___**Muscles developed:** Quadriceps, gluteus maximus, hamstrings.

___**Starting position:** Assume a standing position with a dumbbell in each hand (A) or a barbell across your shoulders and upper back.

___**Eccentric phase:** Inhale as you take a large step forward with one leg. Bend the knee of your forward leg and lower your body until the thigh of the front leg is parallel to the floor (B). (This is essentially a one-leg parallel squat.)

___**Concentric phase:** Exhale as you extend your forward leg, pushing yourself back to your original standing position.

___**Spotting:** Spotting is not necessary if you are doing lunges with dumbbells. If you are doing lunges with a barbell across your back and shoulders, have one spotter stand at each end of the bar. Or perform the lunges into a squat rack that could support the weight in case you cannot return to the standing position.

___**Caution:** Keep your head up and upper body erect throughout the exercise.

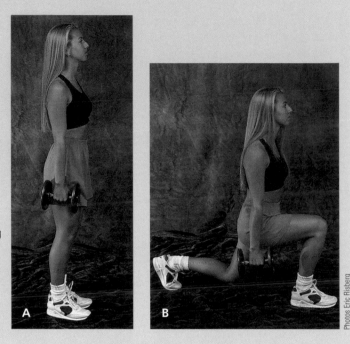

Photos Eric Risberg

Step Up

___**Muscles developed:** Quadriceps, gluteus maximus, hamstrings.

___**Starting position:** Start in a standing position with a dumbbell in each hand (A) or a barbell across your upper back and shoulders.

___**Concentric phase:** Place one foot on the step in front of you. Using your hip and leg muscles, lift yourself up until your leg is straight (B).

___**Eccentric phase:** Lower yourself slowly to the starting position using the same leg.

___**Spotting:** If using dumbbells, you should be all right without a spotter. When using a barbell, have one spotter stand behind you or a spotter at each end of the bar.

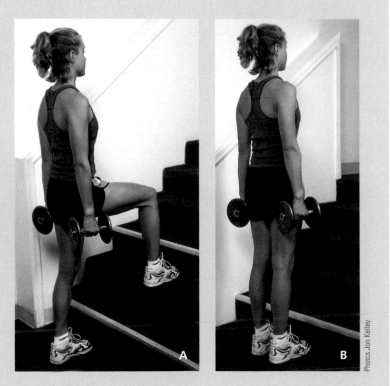

Photos Jon Kelley

Leg Press Machine

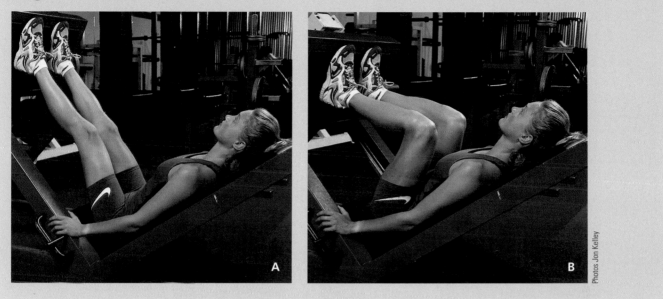

Hack Squat Machine

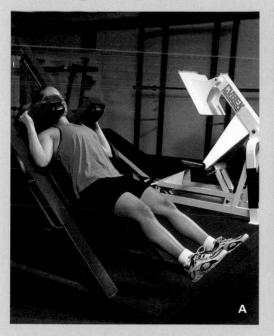
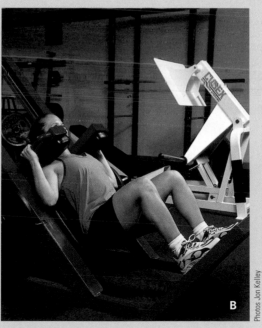

HIP EXTENSION (GLUTEUS MAXIMUS)

Hip Extension Machine

___**Muscles developed:** Gluteus maximus, hamstrings.

___**Starting position:** Start in a standing position with one leg over the padded exercise bar, your hands holding the stability bar, and your hip joint lined up with the point of rotation of the exercise machine (A).

___**Concentric phase:** Exhale as you pull your thigh down and back (hip extension) against the resistance (B).

___**Eccentric phase:** Inhale as you slowly allow your leg to return to the starting position.

___**Additional information:** If you keep your knee bent throughout the exercise, your gluteus maximus muscle will do most of the lifting. If you straighten your knee as you extend your hip, the hamstrings will be in a better position to help with hip extension.

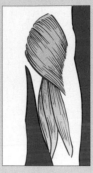

Back

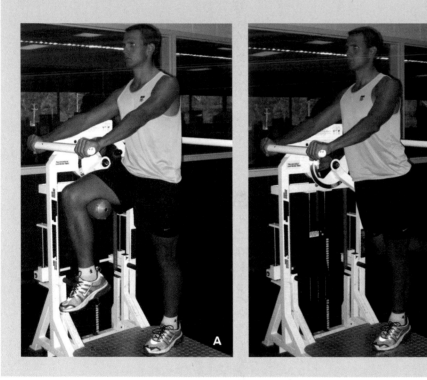

A   B

Photos James Hesson

HIP FLEXION (ILIOPSOAS)

Hip Flexion Machine

___**Muscles developed:** Iliopsoas, rectus femoris.

___**Starting position:** Start in a standing position with one leg against the padded exercise bar and both hands holding the stability bar. The padded exercise bar should be just above your knee joint. Your hip joint should be lined up with the point of rotation of the exercise machine (A).

___**Concentric phase:** Exhale as you pull your bent leg upward against the resistance (B). Tighten your abdominal muscles and keep your lower back flat.

___**Eccentric phase:** Inhale as you lower your leg slowly to the starting position.

___**Caution:** The hip flexors exert a strong pull forward on the lower portion of the spinal column. Therefore, it is important to stabilize the lower spinal column by flexing the abdominal muscles. This exercise is not recommended for individuals with weak abdominal muscles.

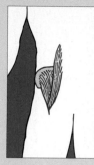

Back

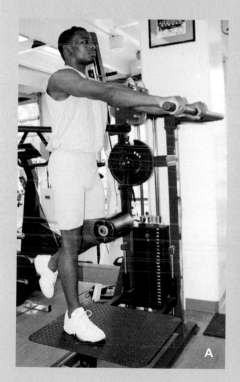

A

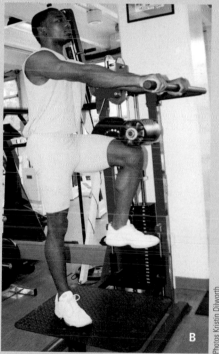

B

Photos Kristin Dilworth

KNEE EXTENSION (QUADRICEPS)

___ **Muscles developed:** Quadriceps.

___ **Starting position:** Start in a seated position with your knees bent and the padded exercise bar in front of your ankle or lower leg. Grasp the handles located on each side of the machine (A).

___ **Concentric phase:** Exhale as you extend your legs at the knee joints (B). Pause at the extended position, but do not go beyond extension.

___ **Eccentric phase:** Inhale as you slowly allow your legs to bend and return to the starting position.

___ **Caution:** Control the exercise movement. Do not hyperextend your knee joint. Do not allow the weight to drop.

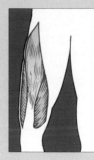

Front

Knee Extension Machine

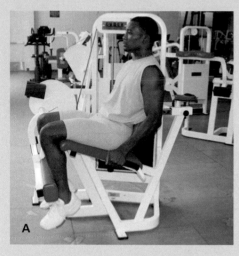

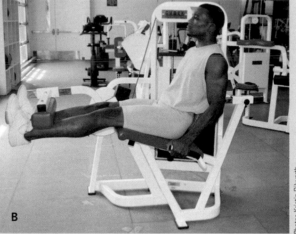

Photos Kristin Dilworth

Knee Extension Machine

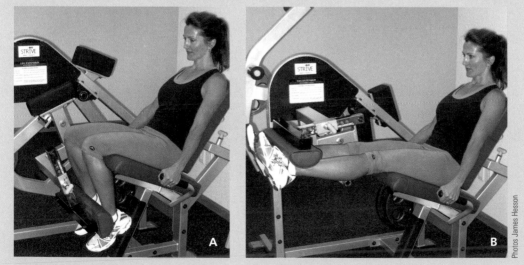

Photos James Hesson

KNEE FLEXION (HAMSTRINGS)

___**Muscles developed:** Hamstrings.

___**Starting position:** Start in a sitting or lying position with your legs straight and the back of your lower leg against the padded exercise bar. Line up your knees with the pivot point of the exercise machine. Grasp the handles. On the seated leg curl, fasten the seat belt to hold your hips in the correct exercise position (A).

___**Concentric phase:** Exhale as you bend your knees and pull your lower legs toward the back of your thighs (B).

___**Eccentric phase:** Inhale as you allow your legs to slowly return to the starting position.

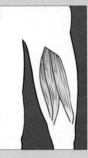

Back

Seated Leg Curl Machine

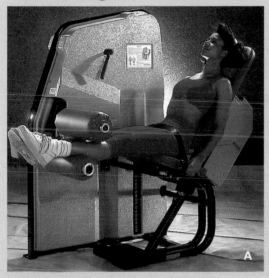

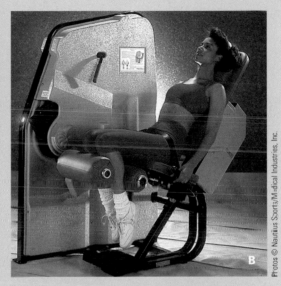

Photos © Nautilus Sports/Medical Industries, Inc.

Lying Leg Curl Machine

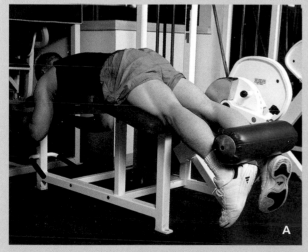

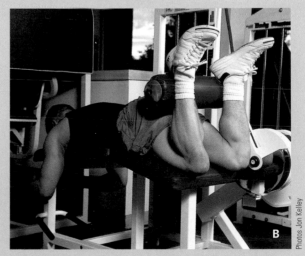

Photos Jon Kelley

ANKLE PLANTAR FLEXION (GASTROCNEMIUS, SOLEUS)

Standing Heel Raise

___**Muscles developed:** Gastrocnemius, soleus.

___**Starting position:** Take a standing position with a barbell across your shoulders and upper back, the front half of both feet elevated so your heels are lower than your toes (A).

___**Concentric phase:** Exhale while moving only at the ankle joint to raise your heels as high as possible (B). Pause briefly and completely contract the muscles on the back of your legs when you are at the highest position you can reach.

___**Eccentric phase:** Inhale as you slowly lower both heels as far as they can go. The best stretch and maximum range of motion are achieved if your heels cannot touch the floor at the bottom position of this exercise.

___**Caution:** Maintaining balance is difficult during this exercise. Performing the exercise in a power rack or on a standing calf-raise machine usually increases the effectiveness of the exercise because it eliminates the balance problem.

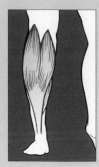

Back

Barbell

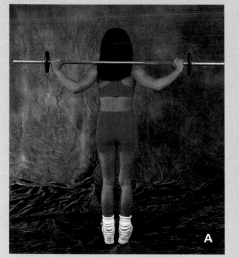

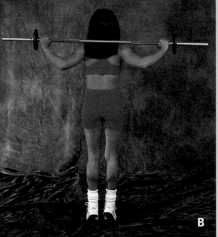

Photos Eric Risberg

Dumbbell

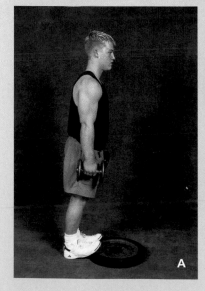

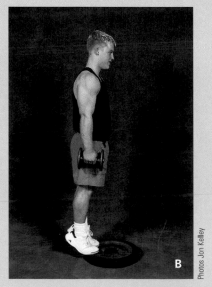

Photos Jon Kelley

Heel Raise Machine

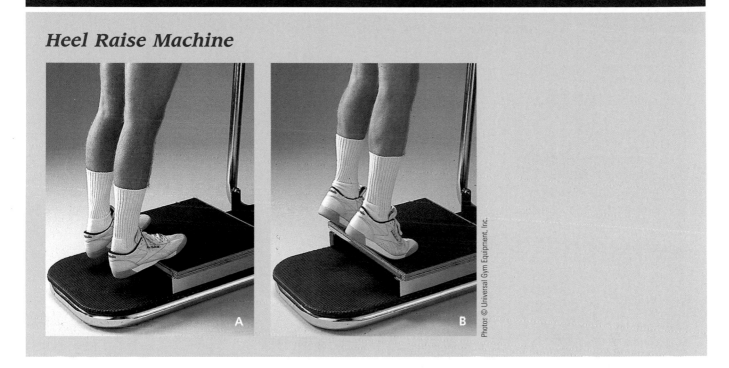

Photos © Universal Gym Equipment, Inc.

Standing Heel Raise Machine

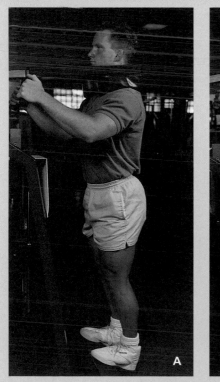 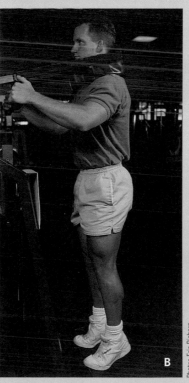

Photos Eric Risberg

One-Dumbbell Heel Raise

___**Muscles developed:**
Gastrocnemius, soleus.

___**Starting position:** Stand with a dumbbell in one hand hanging at arm's length and resting against the side of your thigh. Place all of your body weight on the leg nearest the dumbbell and lift your other foot off the floor (A).

___**Concentric phase:** Exhale as you raise the heel of your support foot as high as possible. Pause at the top.

___**Eccentric phase:** Inhale as you slowly lower the heel of your support foot to a fully stretched position.

___**Additional information:** Place the hand that is not holding the dumbbell on some solid support for balance (B). Use the support hand for balance only; do not pull with that arm to help lift the weight.

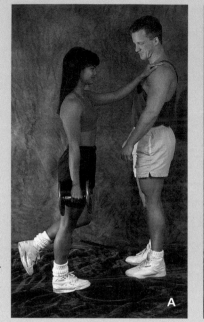
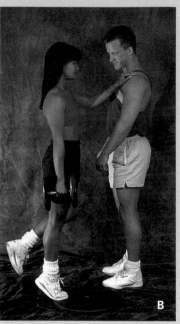

Photos Eric Risberg

Heel Raise on Leg Press Machine

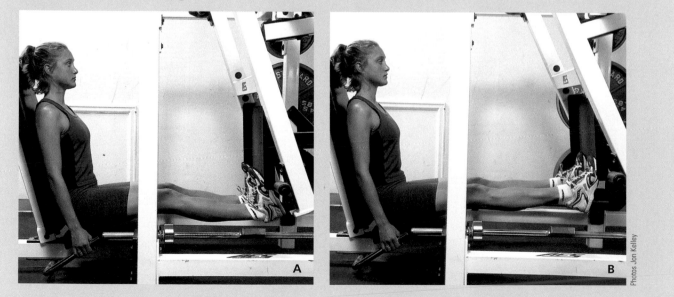

Photos Jon Kelley

Heel Raise on Leg Press Machine

___**Muscles developed:** Gastrocnemius, soleus.

___**Starting position:** Position yourself on a leg press machine. Start with your legs straight, the front half of each foot on the pedals or platform, and your heels lower than the front part of your foot (A).

___**Concentric phase:** Exhale as you press down with the front part of your foot moving only at the ankle joint (B). At the top of your range of motion, hold the muscle contraction and squeeze with your calf muscles.

___**Eccentric phase:** Inhale as you slowly return to the starting position. Stretch the calf muscles in the starting position by allowing the heels to sink as low as possible.

___**Caution:** Do not allow your feet to slip off the pedals or platform.

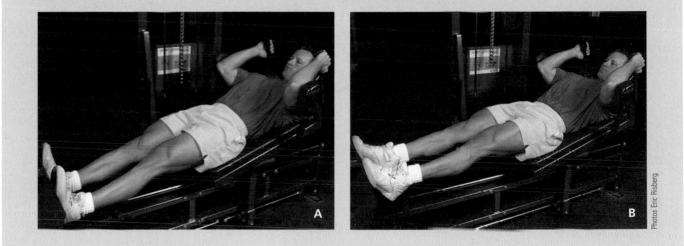

Photos Eric Risberg

Seated Heel Raise

___**Muscles developed:** Soleus (the gastrocnemius becomes much less effective at pulling up on your heel when your knee is bent).

___**Starting position:** Sit with the front half of your foot on the foot plate, your knees under the padded exercise bar and your hands on top of the exercise bar. Your heels should be lower than the front part of your foot (A).

___**Concentric phase:** Lift your heels as high as possible while keeping the front part of your foot on the foot plate (B).

___**Eccentric phase:** Slowly lower your heels to the starting position and stretch.

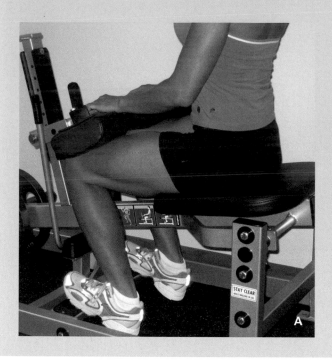

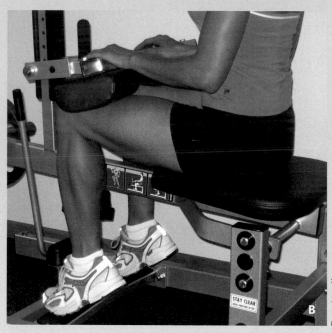

Photos James Hesson

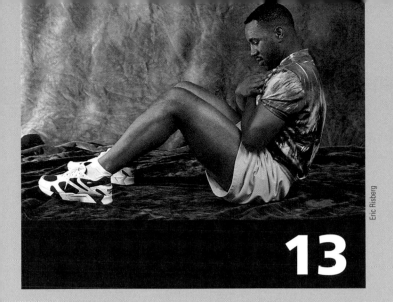
Eric Risberg

13

Trunk Flexion and Extension Exercises

TRUNK FLEXION (ABDOMINALS)

Crunches

___**Muscles developed:** Rectus abdominis and abdominal obliques.

___**Concentric phase:** Exhale as you slowly curl up, lifting your head, neck, shoulders, and upper back off the floor in that order (3 seconds up). Focus on lifting slowly, pulling yourself up with your abdominal muscles. At the upper limit of this movement, crunch (squeeze) your abdominal muscles and hold this fully contracted position (3 seconds hold) while you continue to exhale completely.

___**Eccentric phase:** Slowly release the tension in the abdominal muscles and inhale as you return to the starting position (3 seconds down). Each repetition should take about 9 seconds: 3 seconds up, 3 seconds hold, and 3 seconds down.

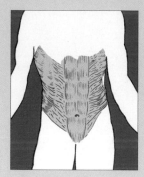

Front

Fingertips on Abs

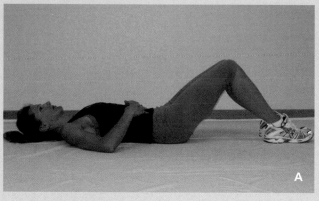

A

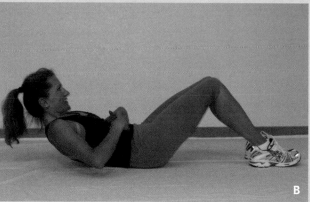

B

Photos James Hesson

Arms Crossed on Chest

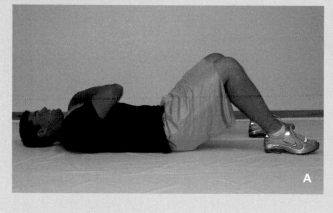

A

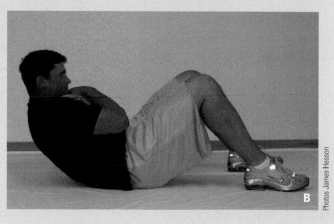

B

Photos James Hesson

Fingertips by Ears

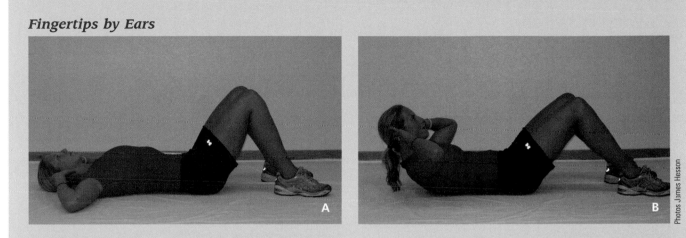

Feet on Bench

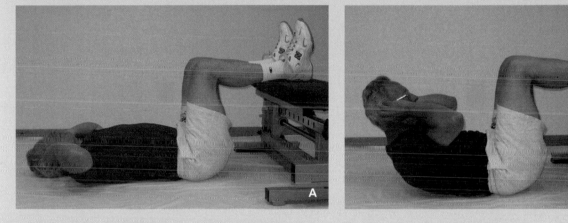

Legs Straight Up

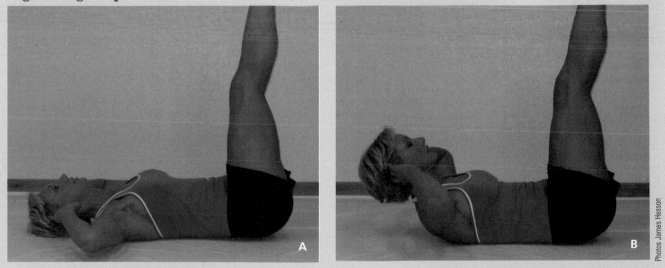

Reverse Crunches

___ **Muscles developed:** Rectus abdominis, abdominal obliques, iliopsoas.

___ **Concentric phase:** Exhale as you slowly pull your legs toward your shoulders (3 seconds). Focusing on the abdominal muscles, pull the pelvic girdle toward the rib cage (B). Hold 3 seconds.

___ **Eccentric phase:** Slowly (3 seconds) return to the starting position and inhale. Each repetition should take about 9 seconds; 3 seconds up, 3 seconds hold, and 3 seconds down.

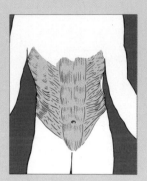

Front

Arms by Sides

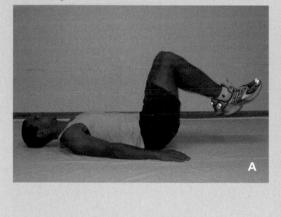

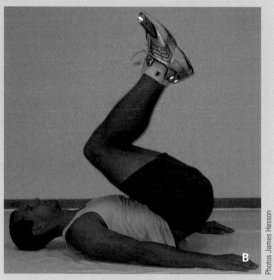

Photos James Hesson

Legs Straight Up

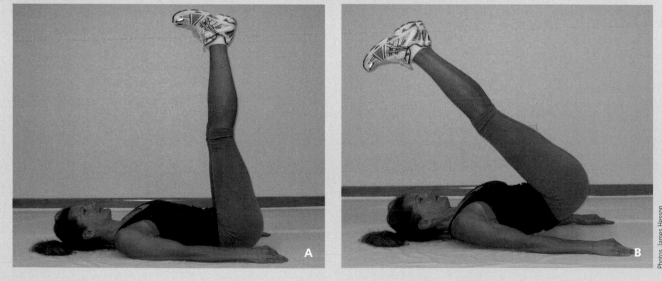

Photos James Hesson

Double Crunch

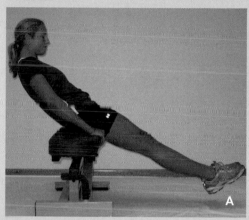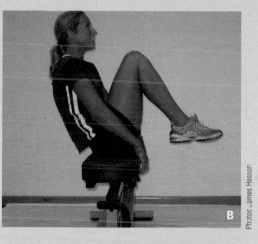

Seated

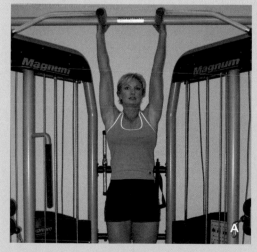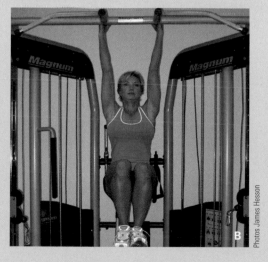

Hanging

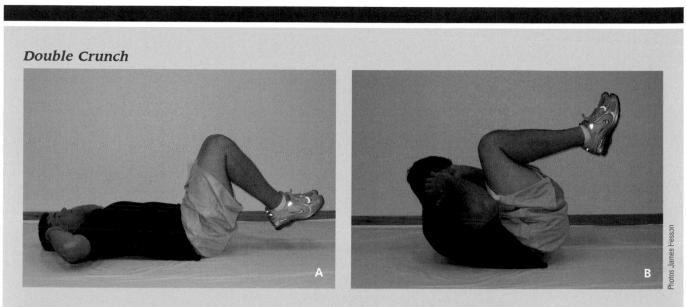

Photos James Hesson

Cross Crunches

Legs to One Side

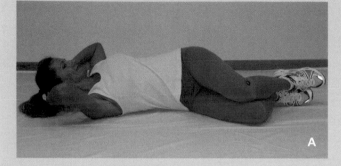

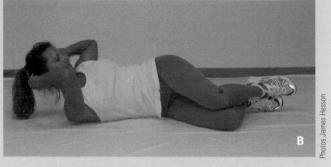

Fingertips on Obliques

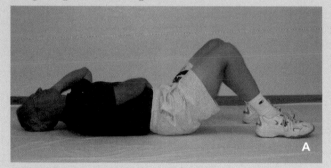

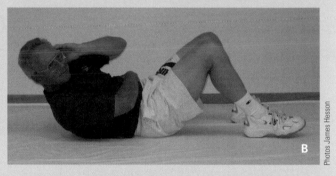

Elbow toward Opposite Knee

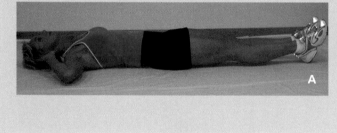

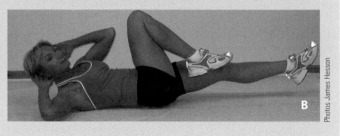

Photos James Hesson

Ab Pull-Ins

___**Muscles developed:** Transverse abdominis.

___**Starting position:** Lying, sitting, standing, or hands and knees.

___**Concentric phase:** Take a deep breath into the chest and then slowly pull the abdomen inward as far as possible (3 seconds). Hold this isometric contraction (3 seconds).

___**Eccentric phase:** Slowly release the tension in the transverse abdominis, exhale, and relax (3 seconds).

Sitting

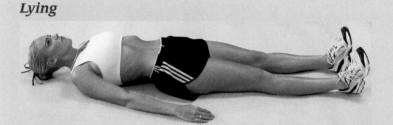

Lying

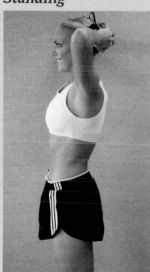

Standing

Hands and Knees

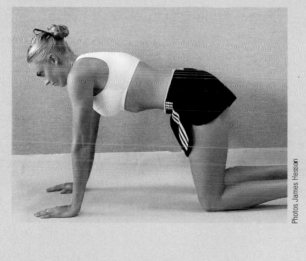

Photos James Hesson

Sit-Ups

___**Muscles developed:** Rectus abdominis, abdominal obliques, iliopsoas, rectus femoris.

___**Starting position:** Start flat on your back with your knees bent and both feet flat on the floor; place your fingertips on the opposite shoulder (A).

___**Concentric phase:** Exhale as you slowly (3 seconds) pull your head, neck, shoulders, upper back, and lower back off the floor, in that order (B). Hold for a 3-second isometric contraction.

___**Eccentric phase:** Slowly (3 seconds) return to the starting position by placing your lower back, upper back, shoulders, neck, and head back on the floor, in that order. Inhale as you near the starting position.

___**Variations:**

1. Twisting sit-ups (require trunk flexion and trunk rotation): Curl up and twist, touching one elbow to the opposite knee. Alternate the direction of the twist on each repetition.

2. Change your arm position to increase or decrease resistance: (a) arms alongside torso, (b) arms crossed on chest, (c) hands beside head, (d) arms extended above head.

3. Add weight. Place it on your upper chest and hold it in place with your hands. When you add weight, you will need to anchor your feet by placing

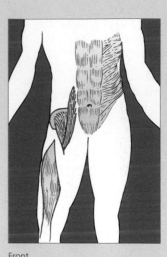

Front

them under something or by having someone hold them.

___**Additional information:** This exercise requires the use of the hip flexors near the end of the concentric phase of the exercise, which does not seem to be a problem if the trunk is fully flexed first. It is okay to strengthen and stretch the hip flexors.

___**Caution:** To avoid low back pain do not pull with the hip flexor muscles until the abdominal muscles are fully contracted.

To avoid neck pain do not pull on your head with your arms.

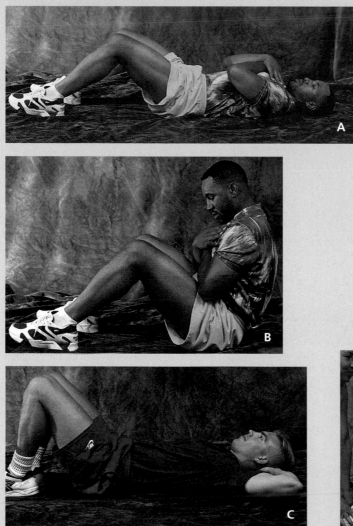

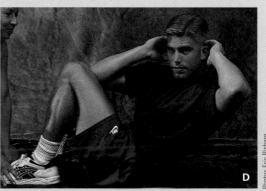

Photos Eric Risberg

Machine Crunches

Abdominal Machine

___ **Muscles developed:** Rectus abdominis, abdominal obliques.

___ **Starting position:** Start in a seated position with your feet under the anchor straps and your upper chest against the padded exercise bar (A).

___ **Concentric phase:** Exhale as you pull with your abdominal muscles to curl your chest toward your hips (B).

___ **Eccentric phase:** Inhale as you slowly allow your chest to return to the starting position.

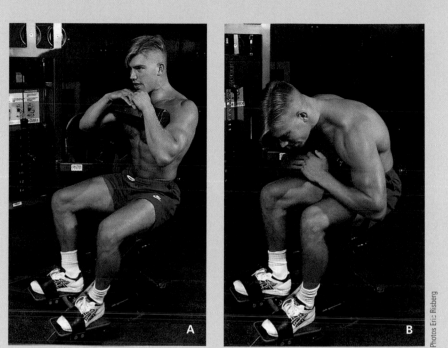

Photos Eric Risberg

Abdominal Crunch Machine

___ **Muscles developed:** Rectus abdominis, abdominal obliques.

___ **Starting position:** Start in a seated position with your upper back against the padded exercise bar. Fasten the seat belt and grasp the handles on the exercise bar.

___ **Concentric phase:** Exhale as you pull with your abdominal muscles to curl your chest toward your hips.

___ **Eccentric phase:** Inhale as you slowly allow your chest to return to the starting position.

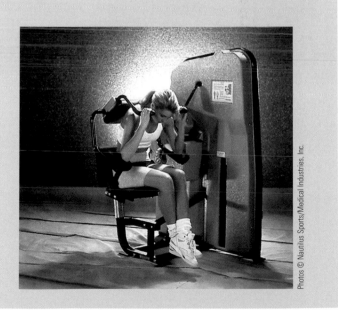

Photos © Nautilus Sports/Medical Industries, Inc.

TRUNK EXTENSION (ERECTOR SPINAE)

Back Extension

___ **Muscles developed:** Erector spinae.

___ **Starting position:** Start on a flat exercise bench with the front of your legs and hips on the bench and with your upper body beyond the end of the bench (A). Have someone hold your feet.

___ **Concentric phase:** Inhale as you slowly raise your upper body to a position in which your back is parallel to the floor (B). Hold 3 seconds.

___ **Eccentric phase:** Exhale as you slowly return to the starting position.

___ **Additional information:** You may use a specially designed back extension bench if you have one available.

___ **Variations:**

1. Place your hands on your lower back with your palms up.

2. Cross your arms on your chest.

3. Place your hands behind your head. As your arms move away from your waist and toward your head, the resistance increases.

4. If you add additional resistance, hold a barbell plate on your chest or behind your head.

___ **Caution:** Perform this exercise in a slow, smooth, and controlled manner. Do not raise your head and shoulders above parallel or arch your back.

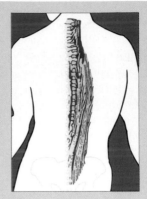

Back

Normal Bench

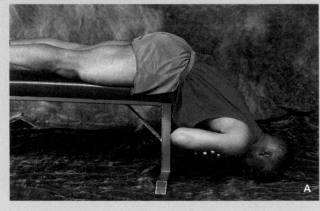

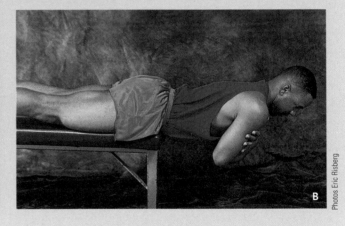

A

B

Photos Eric Risberg

Back Extension Bench

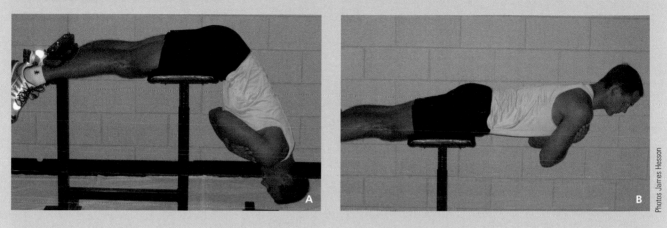

Photos James Hesson

Seated Back Extension Machine

___ **Muscles developed:** Erector spinae.

___ **Starting position:** Start in a seated position leaning forward with your feet on the foot plate. Cross your arms on your chest or place your hands on the front of your thighs (A). Your upper back should be against the padded exercise bar.

___ **Concentric phase:** Inhale as you press backward and extend your back (B).

___ **Eccentric phase:** Exhale as you return slowly to the starting position.

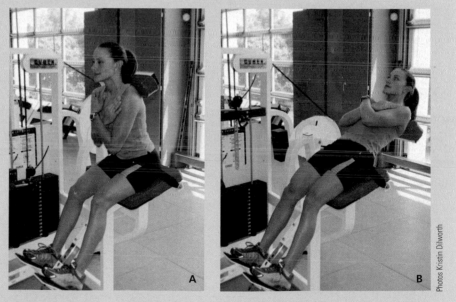

Photos Kristin Dilworth

The Total Ab Solution

A question people frequently ask, while pointing to their protruding abdomen, is, "How can I get rid of this?" If you want to reduce your waist circumference, you will need to work on the following three things. You probably are aware of the first two already, but the last one might surprise you.

1. Reduce your stored body fat.

2. Increase your abdominal muscle strength and muscle tone.

3. Improve your posture.

Reduce

If you have excess body fat on your abdomen, you should

■ Burn more calories than you consume every day.

■ Eat healthy, but eat less than you do now.

■ Increase your aerobic activity to burn more calories per day.

■ Engage in a progressive resistance exercise program (weight training) to build more muscle, burn more calories, and increase your metabolic rate.

Strengthen

Your abdomen might be bulging because of weak abdominal muscles. The earlier part of this chapter contains exercises to strengthen your abdominal muscles.

Posture

If you would like to reduce your waist by 1 or 2 inches immediately, try this: stand up straight, lift your chest, pull your shoulders back, and pull your abdomen in. Poor posture is a major contributing factor for a protruding abdomen. To reinforce good posture, add the following exercises to your regular weight-training program.

1. Perform a back extension exercise to develop the erector spinae muscles, which—as the name implies—cause the spine to be erect and pull the spine into good posture.

2. Perform a rowing exercise with a light weight and concentrate on squeezing your elbows together and pulling your shoulders back in the fully contracted position. Hold this position for 3 seconds and squeeze your shoulder blades together to develop the muscles that pull your shoulders back.

3. Perform deep-breathing straight-arm pull-overs with a light weight to lift and stretch your rib cage.

4. For a few minutes each day, probably in a private place, put a hardbound book on the top of your head and practice standing, sitting, and walking with good posture.

The total Ab solution is a combination of

1. Reducing your stored body fat.

2. Increasing your abdominal muscle strength.

3. Improving your posture.

Before

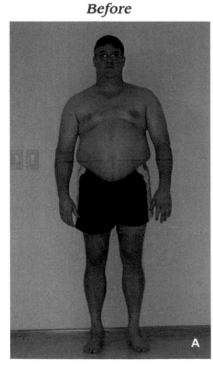

After

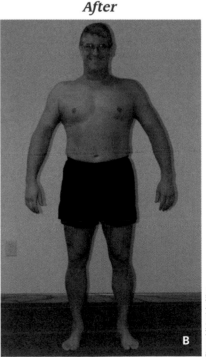

Photos Michael A. Allen

The total Ab Solution: 12 weeks

Back Extension Exercise

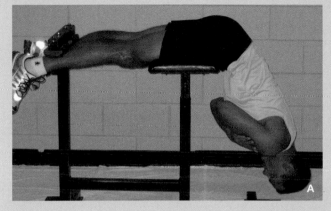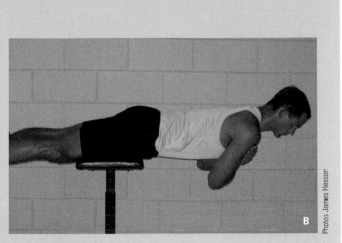

Dumbbell Rowing

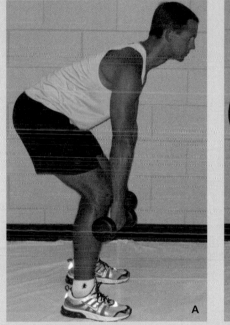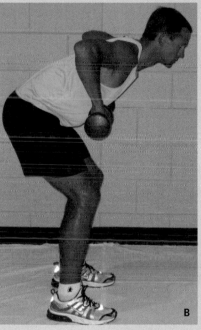

Straight-Arm Pullover

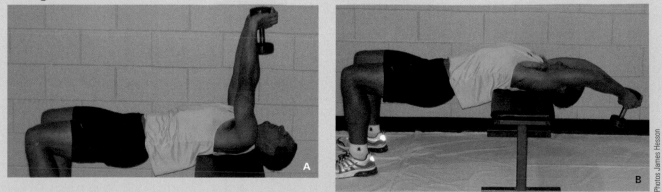

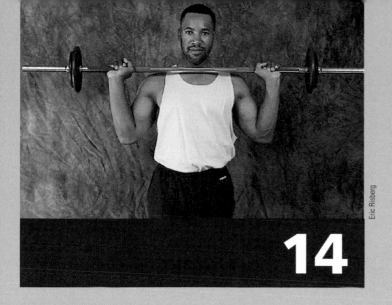

Eric Risberg

14

Measurement and Evaluation

Improving fitness is like taking a trip:

1. You need to know where you are starting (measurements, Chapter 14).

2. You need to decide where you want to go (goals, Chapter 15).

3. You need a plan to get to your destination (exercise plan, Chapter 16; eating plan, Chapter 7).

4. You need to track your progress toward your destination (record keeping, Chapter 14).

5. If you are not going the right direction you need to figure out why (evaluation of progress, Chapter 14).

This chapter covers measurement, record keeping, and evaluation of your progress.

Measurement

Measurements may include strength, muscular endurance, size, body weight, and body fat. Photographs taken before you start training and periodically as you train can provide visual evidence of the changes in your appearance.

Measuring Strength

Strength is the ability of a muscle to exert force. If you are training with weights to gain strength, you can measure your progress in at least two common ways:

1. Workout repetition maximums

2. One-repetition maximums

Weight training for maximum strength gain requires that you lift relatively heavy weight (85 to 100% of your one-repetition maximum) for relatively low repetition maximums (1- to 6-RM). Your **repetition maximum (RM)** is the maximum amount of weight that you can lift for a given number of repetitions. For example, if you can complete 5 repetitions with 155 pounds but cannot do another repetition, your 5-RM is 155 pounds. After a few more workouts, if you can complete 5 repetitions with 160 pounds, you have increased your strength as indicated by the increase in your 5-RM.

Another way to test your progress is by testing your one-repetition maximum (1-RM) periodically using the exercises that you perform in your training program. Your 1-RM is the heaviest weight you can lift one time while maintaining correct exercise technique. You will be limited to the heaviest weight that you can lift through the weakest point in the range of motion. But you will still find the heaviest weight that you can lift one time, and this is a measurement of your ability to exert force (strength).

The first time you test your 1-RM, start with a light weight and perform 10 repetitions to warm up. Then add weight to each subsequent set and perform one repetition in each set until you find the heaviest weight you can lift correctly one time. Try to find your 1-RM within 5 or 6 sets. To find your maximum strength, you need to perform enough sets for the muscles to be warmed up but not so many that the muscles are fatigued.

To perform 1-RM strength tests after the first time, start with a warm-up set of 10 repetitions with 60% of your previous 1-RM. Then perform 1 repetition each at 80%, 85%, 90%, and 95% of your previous 1-RM. After these progressively heavier sets, try for a new personal record based upon how the 95% load felt. If the 95% felt easy, you may want to try 10 pounds more than your previous 1-RM. If the 95% set was very hard, you may want to try just 2½ pounds or 5 pounds more than your previous 1-RM. Rest about 2 minutes between each set and 3 to 5 minutes before attempting your new personal record.

If you fail to maintain correct exercise form on a strength test so that you can lift a heavier weight, you are lying to yourself about your true strength. You also have a greater risk of injury when you attempt to lift a weight heavier than you can really handle. Always use spotters for the exercises in which you could get trapped under a heavy weight.

As a beginning weight trainer, you might want to test 1-RMs once a month for the first 6 to 12 months. After that, increases come more slowly, so testing once every 2 or 3 months might be adequate.

You may choose not to test your 1-RM strength at all. If 1-RM strength is not important, interesting, or motivating to you, you probably have no reason to test it. You need not risk injury or failure attempting 1-RM lifts if it is not important to you.

Measuring Muscular Endurance

Muscular endurance is the ability of a muscle to exert force for a long time or for many repetitions. If you are training with weights to gain muscular endurance, you can measure your progress by performing as many consecutive repetitions as possible with an established weight.

After you warm up, select a weight that is approximately 60% of your 1-RM. Perform as many continuous repetitions as possible without pausing between repetitions. Maintain strict exercise form. Repeat this test once a month, using the same weight every time. An increase in the number of repetitions that you can complete using the same weight is evidence of an increase in your muscle endurance.

Measuring Size

The most common way to measure changes in **muscle size** is to measure the circumference of various body parts using a tape measure. Although circumference measurements include many other kinds of tissue (bone, fat, blood vessels, skin, and so on), muscle and fat are the two tissues that change the most. If you are training your muscles hard and eating properly, circumference gains should be a result of increased muscle, and losses should be a result of decreased fat.

If you measure yourself, you can take measurements anytime you want and take them in the same way every time. A Gulick tape measure is ideal if one is available because it has a spring tension device on the end that enables you to take all measurements with the same tension on the tape. If a Gulick tape is not available, take measurements with a standard cloth tape measure. Place the tape around the circumference so that it is firm but not so tight that the skin is indented. Measure to the nearest ⅛ inch, or ½ centimeter.

Measurements commonly taken by men and women who wish to change their appearance are given here. These represent the circumference measurements that are most likely to change in response to a weight training program. For some body parts, two measurements—relaxed and flexed—are described. If you are trying to lose excess body fat, use the relaxed measurements. If you are trying to gain muscle size, use the flexed measurements. Take the measurements while you are in a standing position with your feet about 6 inches apart. The tape measure should be horizontal unless the directions for a body part specify something different.

Neck *relaxed*: Measure the horizontal circumference midway between your shoulders and head.

Chest *relaxed*: Measure at the largest circumference during relaxed breathing. Do not lift your chest or flex your muscles.

Chest *flexed* (expanded): Measure at the largest circumference of your chest with your lungs filled, rib cage lifted, and muscles flexed.

Waist *relaxed*: Measure the horizontal circumference at the level of your navel. Your abdominal muscles should be in their normal state of tonus for a relaxed standing position.

Waist *flexed*: Measure the horizontal circumference with your abdomen pulled in as far as possible.

Hips *relaxed*: Measure at the largest horizontal circumference.

Hips *flexed*: Tighten your muscles in the hip region, and measure at the largest horizontal circumference.

For all of the following arm and leg measurements, hold the tape perpendicular to the limb segment being measured. Measure both arms and both legs.

Thigh *relaxed*: Measure the horizontal circumference midway between your hip joint and your knee joint.

Thigh *flexed*: Slightly bend your knee joint and contract all of your thigh muscles. Measure midway between your hip joint and knee joint.

Calf or leg *relaxed*: Measure at the largest circumference.

Calf or leg *flexed*: Measure the largest circumference with the muscles of your leg flexed.

Upper arm *relaxed*: With your arms hanging relaxed, measure your horizontal circumference midway between the shoulder joint and the elbow joint.

Upper arm *flexed*: Raise your arm to shoulder height. Bend your elbow and flex all muscles of your upper arm. Measure the largest circumference.

Forearm *relaxed*: With your arm hanging in a normal relaxed position, measure the largest circumference of your forearm, between the wrist and the elbow.

Forearm *flexed*: Bend your elbow and wrist so that as many forearm muscles as possible can be contracted. Measure at the largest circumference between your wrist and elbow.

All these measurements should be taken the first time you measure. After that you may choose to measure just the ones in which you are most interested. Weight trainers might want to measure once a month. How often you measure is up to you. It is your training program.

The measurements suggested here are ones that are commonly used. Because they are used to measure your progress—muscle gain or fat loss—they should be taken exactly the same way each time and, if possible, with the same tape measure. These measurements are taken to provide information about the effectiveness of your training program.

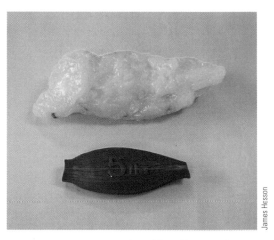

Models: (top) 5 pounds of fat; (bottom) 5 pounds of muscle

Measuring Body Weight

If your goal is to change your **body weight,** this can be measured on an accurate scale. It is best to use the same scale, at the same time of day, wearing as little clothing as possible and the same clothing each time. A scale measures your total body weight but does not differentiate between muscle and fat. Muscle is more dense than fat. As you gain muscle and lose fat, you may lose inches but not pounds.

Estimating Body Fat

The percentage of your total body weight that is stored as body fat, called **percent body fat,** can be measured in many ways. All methods have advantages and disadvantages, and many factors can affect the accuracy of body fat estimates. You should keep in mind that this measurement is an estimate, with an error range.

Rather than estimating percent body fat, you can have **skinfold measurements** taken at the sites where you are most interested in losing excess subcutaneous body fat. If they are taken by someone who is trained and experienced, skinfold measurements can be highly accurate. A reduction in your skinfold measurement at a given site is an indication of a loss of stored subcutaneous body fat at that site.

Photographs

Changes in appearance take place gradually and cannot be seen as they occur. Taking photographs of various poses can be an excellent means of periodically checking your progress. A photograph is a good way see yourself as you really are. The photograph should be taken while you are wearing as little clothing as possible, such as a swimsuit. Subsequent photographs should be taken with the same camera, location, position, and distance. Photographs taken before you start training can be highly motivating, and they are fun to have after you have gotten into better shape.

Record Keeping

Record each training session. Write down what you do during each workout immediately after you do it.

Weight training is not an exact science. Although weight training adheres to some general guidelines, many variables affect your progress. Each individual is different and responds differently to a weight training stimulus. The information you record during your training sessions can be a valuable source of information about your personal response to a variety of weight training exercises. From this, you will be able to look back through your

Monday,
September 23, 2010
Bench Press
135 lbs. x 10 reps
155 lbs. x 8 reps
175 lbs. x 6 reps

Figure 14.1 Open-page log

records and compare your progress using various training methods and exercises. This will help you find which exercises and training methods work best for you. The important things to record are

■ Name of each exercise.

■ Order in which exercises are performed.

■ Resistance used in each set.

■ Repetitions completed in each set.

■ Day of the week.

■ Date.

■ A general comment about how you felt or anything that might have influenced your training that day, positive or negative (for example, "felt tired, 2 hours sleep").

Keeping track of your weight training sessions helps provide motivation and ensure the correct exercise stimulus. From the written record of what you were able to do during the previous training session comes a challenge to do a little bit more—one more repetition or 5 more pounds. Figures 14.1 and 14.2 provide examples of written record

keeping—the first informal and the second a printed form.

Evaluation of Progress

Physical changes take time. Changes usually appear faster in beginners than more experienced exercisers. How often you measure to evaluate your progress is up to you. It is your training program. You are in control.

Genetic Potential

Each individual has some upper limit to the amount of strength or size or muscle endurance that he or she can gain. For the beginning weight trainer, gains are relatively easy and fast. As progress continues and gains get close to a person's **genetic limit,** the gains become more difficult and slower.

One of the most intriguing aspects of weight training is that you have no way of knowing when you have reached your genetic limit or if *anyone* has ever reached his or her limit. After years of weight training, bodybuilders and

strength athletes continue to improve, though the rate of improvement slows.

Problem Solving

It you have not made progress for a long time (2 or 3 months), problem solving is in order. What might be the cause of your lack of progress? Change the one thing that you think is most likely causing your lack of progress. Allow 3 or 4 weeks for the change to start making a difference. If you have not progressed after a month, try changing a different variable. Give it time to work.

Changing more than one variable at a time may leave you with more questions than answers. Changing too often (less than 4 to 6 weeks) might not allow enough time to find out what works for you and what does not. Keep in mind that what works for you now may not work when your body adapts to it. Some of the factors to consider in solving a lack of progress in weight training are

■ Amount of resistance.

■ Number of repetitions.

■ Number of sets.

■ Rest between sets.

■ Number of exercises per body part.

■ Total number of exercises performed.

■ Order of exercises.

■ Frequency of training.

■ Concentration when exercising.

■ Intensity of training.

■ Regularity of training—hour and day.

■ Motivation level.

■ Nutrition.

■ Rest.

■ Other activities.

■ Mental stress.

■ Drugs.

■ Alcohol.

■ Tobacco.

STRENGTH AND MUSCULAR ENDURANCE PROGRESS LOG (EXAMPLE)

Name _____ Section _____

Exercise	Date 23 Sept 2010 Wt	Rep	Wt	Rep	Wt	Rep	Wt	Rep	Wt	Rep	Wt	Rep	Wt	Rep
Bench Press	135	10												
	155	8												
	175	6												
Rowing	135	10												
	155	8												
	175	6												
Overhead Press	60	10												
	80	8												
	100	6												
BB Curl	40	10												
	60	8												
	80	6												
Squat	135	10												
	185	8												
	235	6												
DB Calf Raise	BW+10	10												
	BW+15	8												
	BW+20	6												
Ab Crunch	BW	10												
		10												
Back Ext.	BW	10												
		10												
		10												

Figure 14.2 Sample form for record keeping

Name _____ Section _____

Size Measurement

Directions

Read the discussion on Measuring Size in Chapter 14.

	1st Measurement Date:	2nd Measurement Date:	3rd Measurement Date:	4th Measurement Date:
Height ⟶				
Weight ⟶				
Neck (relaxed) ⟶				
Chest (relaxed) ⟶				
(flexed) ⟶				
Waist (relaxed) ⟶				
(flexed) ⟶				
Hips (relaxed) ⟶				
(flexed) ⟶				

Right (R) Left (L)	R	L	R	L	R	L	R	L
Thigh (relaxed) ⟶								
(flexed) ⟶								
Calf (relaxed) ⟶								
(flexed) ⟶								
Upper Arm (relaxed) ⟶								
(flexed) ⟶								
Forearm (relaxed) ⟶								
(flexed) ⟶								

Name _____   Section _____

Strength Measurement

Directions

1. Read the section Measuring Strength in Chapter 14.

2. Train with weights for at least 2 weeks before testing your strength.

3. Test your strength every 4 weeks after the first test.

4. Move the weight in a smooth, continuous manner.

5. Maintain strict exercise form.

6. Do not hold your breath.

7. Increase the weight for each set.

8. Rest between sets.

9. Rest 3 to 5 minutes before your final record attempt.

10. Start with a light weight that you can lift 10 times. After that first warm-up set, continue increasing the weight and performing one repetition until you reach your one-repetition maximum (1-RM). Try to reach your 1-RM within 5 or 6 total sets.

11. Record the date, the exercise, and your 1-RM.

12. Always remember "**Safety First.**" Don't injure yourself attempting 1-RM lifts.

Strength Test	1st Test	2nd Test	3rd Test	4th Test
	Date:	Date:	Date:	Date:
Exercise	Weight	Weight	Weight	Weight

Name _____ Section _____

Muscle Endurance Measurement

Directions

1. Read the section on Measuring Muscular Endurance in Chapter 14.

2. Test your strength to find your one-repetition maximum.

3. Select a weight that is approximately 60% of your 1-RM.

4. After you warm up, perform as many continuous repetitions as possible, with absolutely no pause to rest between repetitions.

5. Move the weight in a smooth, controlled manner.

6. Maintain strict exercise form.

7. Test your muscle endurance every 4 weeks after the first test.

8. Use the same weight for each exercise every time that you test yourself for muscle endurance on that exercise. An increase in repetitions using the same weight should indicate an increase in muscle endurance.

9. Always remember "**Safety First.**" Don't injure yourself.

Muscle Endurance Test		1st Test	2nd Test	3rd Test	4th Test
		Date:	Date:	Date:	Date:
Exercise	Weight	Reps	Reps	Reps	Reps

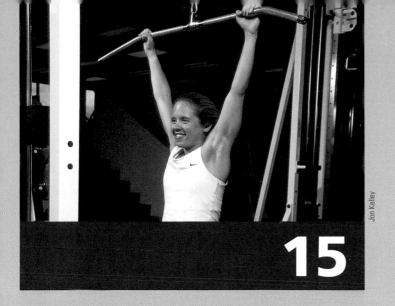
Jon Kelley

15

A Formula for Success

"Success" has a different meaning for each of us. In this chapter, **success** is defined as **setting a goal and achieving it.** Successful people achieve the goals that they have set for themselves. A successful person reaches big success as a result of many smaller successes. Success breeds success. Achieving smaller goals that lead to larger ones is important. This process results in a lifestyle that is as enjoyable as the attainment of each goal. People with goals are people with a passion for living. People with goals have decided what they want out of life and they are going after it. They live with passion and direction.

A Formula for Success
Written Goals

Goals are an extremely important part of any successful weight training program. Putting the necessary effort into weight training is difficult without some desirable goal to be reached. **A successful weight training program cannot be planned without a goal.** All successful training programs are based on a desired outcome. If you don't have a desired outcome, how can you plan to reach it?

Goals should be as specific as possible. This may be difficult if you are just beginning a new activity such as weight training, but try to be as specific as possible.

Decide on a goal and write it down. This is an important step. Make a contract with yourself. Thoughts and spoken words become modified with the passing of time, but your written goal will remain the same every time you read it.

Once you have written your goal, you may begin to steer a course rather than drift aimlessly. Knowing where you want to go, before and during your journey, is critical to reaching your destination.

After you have a clearly defined written goal you can make decisions quickly and easily. When you know exactly where you are going you can decide quickly; "Yes, this will take me in the right direction" or "No, this will take me in the wrong direction."

To obtain great success or achievement, goals must take into consideration your unique individual qualities. Don't set yourself up for failure. Your goals should be challenging but attainable. They need to be based on where you are starting and what you believe is possible.

Most people find happiness in striving for and attaining worthwhile goals. Boredom is often the result of not having goals. Some say weight training is boring or life is boring.

People who are bored are probably not working toward goals that they are passionate about. If you know what you want, weight training and life become exciting adventures—not easy, but certainly not boring. When people stop striving for goals, they stop growing.

Positive Thinking

Positive thinking is such an essential ingredient in success that some people have identified it as the only ingredient. One reason is the goal-setting stage is primarily a private process that others do not see. Positive thinking, by contrast, is obvious to everyone who comes in contact with the person.

Your subconscious mind works on what you feed it. One sure way to block success is to set a goal and not believe that you can achieve it. Instead, fill your mind with positive thoughts, send out positive thoughts, and resist the negative thoughts of others. Positive people see the good side of bad situations and the bright side of every situation. Is a half glass of water half full or half empty? Your answer to that simple question may reveal a lot about your attitude. Many people dwell on what they don't have and can't do while others focus on what they do have and can do.

Don't strive for success without happiness. This would be an unfulfilling success. Truly successful people enjoy what they are doing. Most people are as happy as they decide to be. Your happiness is based on your internal reaction to external events.

Imagination is a stronger force than willpower. Form a clear detailed image of what you want. Every creation starts with an idea. You become what you think about. If you focus on failure, you will fail. If you focus on success, you will succeed. Positive thoughts create positive results.

Desire is the power behind human action. Successful people have an all-consuming, burning desire to reach their goals.

Positive thinking includes belief. Belief is more than wishing—it is knowing without a doubt that you can achieve your goal.

The Subconscious Mind

The subconscious mind is extremely powerful, and it can help solve your problems. The subconscious mind works day and night to bring about what you imagine or visualize. The subconscious mind is the reason why positive thinking is so important. If you expect to fail, you will fail. If you expect to succeed, you will succeed.

Your subconscious mind can be programmed through repetition. Repetition can accomplish great tasks. Therefore, you should read your goals aloud at least twice each day, morning and night. Read your goals before each training session so you know why you are there and what you need to do.

You have an opportunity to participate in your own creation. You can become what you want to become. You can be the person you want to be.

Use your subconscious mind, use autosuggestion, and repeat your goal to yourself regularly. Once an idea is deeply embedded in your subconscious mind, it will go to work to help you achieve your goal.

Keep a notepad and pencil handy for ideas. Solutions will come to you.

Write these ideas immediately, so you can expand on them later. Often, if these ideas are not written down immediately, they are gone. You may remember that you had a great idea but not be able to remember what it was.

A Written Plan

Everyone has the same amount of time each week, 168 hours. Why do some people accomplish more than others? They learn to manage themselves and use their time wisely. Lack of time indicates a lack of organization. Some people say they don't have time to exercise. What they should say is that exercise is less important to them than anything else they do.

Effectiveness is doing the right things. This requires a **focus on *results.*** Your time should be spent on things that make a difference. In your weight training program, be sure that you are doing the things that lead to the achievement of your goal. Don't waste your time on things that don't matter.

Efficiency is doing things right. This requires a **focus on *methods.*** Once you are doing the right exercises and you are doing the exercises right, you will be on your way to reaching your goals.

Plan time to continue learning about weight training. The more you learn, the better you can plan to reach your goals.

Take time to plan how you will reach your goals. Evaluate your progress toward your goals. After evaluation, make the necessary adjustments in your plan.

Do It!

All the previous steps are useless unless you do it. People of action control the world. You never get anywhere unless you move. Decide what activities will lead to your goals and then act upon your decision. Learn to act and make things happen instead of reacting to things that happen.

Work and sacrifice are required to reach your goals. There is always a price to pay for anything worthwhile.

Steps in the Formula for Success

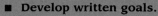

- **Develop written goals.**
  - Set short-term goals that you can achieve that will lead to your long-term goals.
  - Fix in your mind exact, measurable goals.
  - Write your goals.
- **Use positive thinking.**
  - Believe that you can reach your goals.
  - Have faith in your ability to achieve your goals.
- **Use your subconscious mind.**
  - Read your goals aloud at least twice each day, morning and night.
- Read your weight training goals before each training session.
- **Develop a written plan.**
  - Take time to plan, so your efforts are directed toward your goals.
  - Evaluate your progress and modify your plan.
- **Do it.**
  - Start working toward your goal and don't stop until you reach it.
  - Enjoy the journey as much as the arrival.

Poorly Written Goals	Well-Written Goals
Increase my bench press. *(no set amount, no time limit)*	I will bench press 240 pounds one time by _____. *(day, month, year)*
Firm up my muscles. *(too general; how will you know?)*	I will perform 30 repetitions of the barbell curl using 60 pounds by _____. *(day, month, year)*
Get in shape. *(too general; how will you measure this?)*	I will have a 28-inch waist by _____. *(day, month, year)*

Table 15.1 Examples of Poor Goals and Good Goals

You always have to pay the price in advance. Don't expect to get something for nothing. You must work at success. Once you have decided what must be done, discipline yourself to do it.

One of the most common reasons for failure is failure to take action. Procrastination has caused more failure than any other single factor. Now is the time to take action. The clock of your life is running, and it cannot be stopped or reversed. There are no time-outs.

Once you get started, you must persist. *Persistence* is a familiar word but a rare quality. Many who take the first step fail because they do not continue working toward their goal. Stick with it, don't give up, never give up. If your goal is worthwhile, it is worth your best effort.

This formula for success will work for almost anything you want. It is presented in this book to help you reach your weight training goals.

Writing Weight Training Goals

Your goals must be **believable,** achievable, reasonable, and attainable (Table 15.1). Don't set yourself up for failure. A goal to bench press 1000 pounds by the end of this year is not believable. A goal to lose 20 pounds of fat by the end of this week is not believable. Set motivating goals that you can sincerely believe in. After you reach this goal, you can set another believable goal. Success breeds success.

Goals must be **compatible.** Running a marathon (26.2 miles) in less than 2 hours and performing a 1 repetition maximum squat with 1000 pounds on the same day are not compatible training goals.

Your weight training goals must be **specific, measurable,** and **motivat-**

ing. You must set a **specific time limit,** a date when you will reach your goal.

"Get in shape" is not a goal statement. It is not specific or measurable. "I will have a 32-inch waist by December 15, 2010" is specific, measurable, and motivating if you want a 32-inch waist. "Get stronger" is not a goal statement. "I will squat 185 pounds one time by May 15, 2010" is specific, measurable, and motivating if you want to squat 185 pounds.

Complete the "Goal Setting" assignment at the end of this chapter. If you have too many goals at one time, you may not be able to reach them all.

Rather than setting too many goals at one time, focus on a few goals that are most important to you. However, you may have several short-term body measurement goals that are compatible and lead to the same long-term goal. Or you could have several short-term strength goals that lead to the same long-term goal.

The goals you set must be **your own personal goals,** not someone else's goals for you. They must be *your* goals, something *you* want, for them to be motivating.

If you do not want to increase your muscular strength, muscular size, or muscular endurance; if you do not want to perform better, look better, or feel better; if you cannot think of any motivating goal that weight training can help you achieve— you will probably perceive weight training to be difficult, time-consuming, and boring.

If you want to improve your muscular strength, muscular size, or muscular endurance; if you want to perform better, look better, or feel better; if you have a motivating goal that weight training can help you achieve—you will perceive weight training to be worthwhile and interesting.

Name _____ Section _____

Goal Setting

Directions

1. Read Chapter 15, "A Formula for Success."

2. Set weight training goals that are specific, measurable, believable, and compatible.

3. Set a specific date by which you will reach your goals.

4. Set goals that create a burning desire within you. These must be your goals. They must be something you want very much. They must be motivating goals. The greater your desire for a goal, the greater will be your chance of achieving it.

5. Set goals for measurable changes in muscular strength or size or endurance.

6. Write at least one, but no more than three, personal weight training goals. These should be short-term goals that can be reached in the next 3 months.

Goal 1: I will _____

_____

by _____
(day, month, year)

Is this goal specific? ____ Measurable? ____ Believable? ____ Compatible? ____ Motivating? ____

Have you set a specific date when you will reach this goal? ____

Goal 2: I will _____

_____

by _____
(day, month, year)

Is this goal specific? ____ Measurable? ____ Believable? ____ Compatible? ____ Motivating? ____

Have you set a specific date when you will reach this goal? ____

Goal 3: I will _____

_____

by _____
(day, month, year)

Is this goal specific? ____ Measurable? ____ Believable? ____ Compatible? ____ Motivating? ____

Have you set a specific date when you will reach this goal? ____

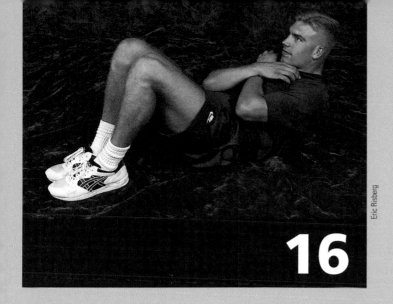

Eric Risberg

16

Planning Your Personal Weight Training Program

This chapter is designed to guide you through the process of designing your own personal weight training program. It also includes a review of basic weight training principles, suggested lifetime weight training programs, a simple home weight training program, time management suggestions, and study suggestions for students.

Basic Weight Training Principles

Three basic principles underlying all weight training progress are specificity, overload, and progression.

Specificity

You must exercise the specific muscles that you want to develop. You also must follow specific exercise guidelines to produce the specific type of change that you want: muscle strength, muscle size, or muscle endurance.

Overload

The overload principle is the basis of all training programs. In weight training, *overload* means a muscle must be forced to work harder than normal.

Progression

Once your muscles adapt to a given workload, it is no longer an overload. The workload must be progressively increased as the muscle adapts to each new demand. This is the principle of progression.

Considerations in Planning Your Weight Training Program

Your Goals

Planning a weight training program must begin with your goals. You can train for three basic aspects of muscle fitness:

1. Muscle strength
2. Muscle size
3. Muscle endurance

Any weight training program that you choose will result in some increase in all three areas. Untrained beginners gain on almost any weight training program as long as progressive overload is applied. Some general guidelines have emerged from research and experience, and they will help you focus on developing the aspect of most interest to you.

Which Exercises?

Which exercises are the best? The best weight training exercises are **compound exercises.** These exercises require more than one joint or muscle to move the weight. With compound exercises, such as the squat and the bench press, large amounts of muscle are exercised at the same time. Exercises that require both arms or both legs to work together allow the use of more weight and maintain a balance of development on both sides of the body.

All weight trainers use the same basic exercises. Some of these exercises are included in the basic weight training program in this book.

Choose exercises for your training program with overall development in mind. Developing the entire body is better than ignoring certain body parts or overdeveloping one or two body parts. As you select your exercises, keep balanced development in mind. Both sides of your body should be developed equally, and opposing muscles or muscle groups should always be exercised.

In the beginning, if you don't know the muscles, remember that for every exercise action or movement you perform there should be an opposite action or movement in another exercise. For example, if you perform an exercise that develops the elbow flexors, you should also do an exercise that develops elbow extensors.

Number of Exercises

One exercise per body part is enough for the beginning weight trainer. One exercise for each major muscle group or body part will result in about 8 to 12 basic exercises in your training program.

Order of Exercises

Exercise your largest muscles first and work your way down to your smallest muscles last. The largest muscles require the most energy and need the smaller muscles to assist. If your smaller muscles are fatigued first, you will have difficulty handling enough weight to exercise your larger muscles. For example, most back exercises require grip strength. If your finger and forearm flexors have already been exercised, they will fatigue before your larger stronger back muscles. Your largest muscles are located on your torso. Proceeding outward on the arms and legs, the muscles get smaller.

The order of exercises may also be based on a *work–rest principle.* If a muscle is worked during an exercise, it is allowed to rest during the next exercise. If you are exercising opposing muscle groups, you may work a muscle and then let it rest as you work on the opposing muscle. This allows you to complete more work in less time.

Another consideration in the order of exercises is whether to perform a circuit or to do the exercises in a traditional noncircuit manner. When you perform a circuit, you do each exercise in your training program once in a specified order. Then you perform each exercise again and possibly again in that same order. The traditional way of lifting weights is to do all of the sets of one exercise before moving to the next exercise.

Resistance

The amount of weight that you use depends on what you want to develop. The general rule is that for *strength* you need a heavier weight and few repetitions. For muscle *endurance,* you need a lighter weight and more repetitions. Muscle *size* (body shaping and toning) development is in-between, using moderate weight and repetitions. Before using heavier weights, complete warm-up sets with lighter weights.

Muscle strength: 85 to 100% of 1 RM or 1 to 6 RM (repetition maximum)

Muscle size: 70 to 85% of 1 RM or 6 to 12 RM

Muscle endurance: 50 to 70% of 1 RM or 12 to 20(+) RM

Starting Weight

Begin with a weight that is light so that you can perform each exercise correctly. Increase the resistance gradually. Don't be in a big hurry to increase resistance. If you give your body time to adapt, you will experience more progress, less muscle soreness, fewer injuries, less frustration, and more enjoyment. You have plenty of time to add resistance if you are *weight training for life.*

Repetitions

The resistance that you choose will affect the repetitions you can perform.

Muscle strength: 1 to 6 reps

Muscle size: 6 to 12 reps

Muscle endurance: 12 to 20+ reps

Sets

The resistance and repetitions influence the number of sets that you perform for each exercise. Start with a low number of sets and gradually increase the number of sets as your body adapts to each new workload. This is progressive overload.

Muscle strength: 4 to 8 sets

Muscle size: 3 to 6 sets

Muscle endurance: 2 to 4 sets

Rest between Sets

Your goals, resistance, repetitions, and sets determine the amount of rest between sets.

Muscle strength, heavy resistance, low repetitions, multiple heavy sets: Rest 2 to 4 minutes between sets.

	Muscle Strength	Muscle Size	Muscle Endurance	Muscle Tone
Resistance	85 to 100% of 1-RM	70 to 85% of 1-RM	50 to 70% of 1-RM	60 to 80% of 1-RM
Repetitions	1 to 6 RM	6 to 12 RM	12 to 20(+) RM	8 to 12 RM
Sets	4 to 8	3 to 6	2 to 4	1 to 3
Rest (between sets)	2 to 4 minutes	1 to 2 minutes	30 to 90 seconds	30 to 60 seconds

Table 16.1 Summary of Weight Training Guidelines

Muscle size, moderate resistance, moderate repetitions, multiple sets: Rest 1 to 2 minutes between sets.

Muscle endurance, light resistance, high repetitions, fewer sets: Rest 30 to 90 seconds between sets.

Table 16.1 provides a summary of the weight training guidelines outlined above.

Frequency

A muscle usually requires at least 2 or 3 days of rest to recover and adapt before it should be exercised again. Exercising a muscle 3 days per week with 48 to 72 hours of rest between training sessions works well for most beginning weight trainers.

Advanced weight trainers perform different exercises on different days. They may exercise 4, 5, or 6 days a week, but they do not exercise the same body parts each day or the same muscles on two consecutive days.

Fixed or Variable Exercise Load

A load is applied to each exercise in two basic ways: fixed or variable. With a **fixed load,** the resistance, repetitions, sets, and rest interval remain the same (fixed) during a single training session.

Example: Bench Press

150 pounds

10 reps

3 sets

1 minute rest between sets

With a **variable load,** the resistance, repetitions, and rest interval change for each set of an exercise during a single training session.

Example: Bench Press

150 pounds, 10 reps, 1 minute rest

170 pounds, 8 reps, 2 minutes rest

190 pounds, 6 reps, 3 minutes rest

210 pounds, 4 reps, 4 minutes rest

Progression

Some general rules are helpful in applying the progression principle to the overload:

Change only one variable at a time (resistance, repetitions, sets, rest).

Increase reps or sets before increasing resistance.

Decrease reps when increasing resistance.

Decrease the rest interval between sets to increase muscular endurance.

Muscle Tone or Muscle Fitness

Beginners often say they just want to tone their muscles. They are not interested in developing strength, size, or endurance. What is muscle tone? When the word *tone* is used in reference to muscle tissue, it refers to muscle tissue that is firm, sound, and resilient. This is in contrast to the loose, flabby, and weak muscles of a sedentary person. Although developing muscle tone is desirable, measuring changes in muscle tone is difficult.

When you train for strength, size, or endurance, an improvement in **muscle tone** will occur. If you train for **muscle tone,** you will experience improvement in strength, size, and muscle endurance. The following are some guidelines for those who wish to train for muscle tone.

60 to 80% of 1-RM

8 to 12 reps

1 to 3 sets of each exercise

30 to 60 seconds rest between sets

3 days per week (every other day)

Although training for muscle tone is possible, the lack of measurable progress can result in a loss of motivation. How will you know if you are getting more tone? How much more tone do you have this week than last week? Therefore, beginning weight trainers are advised to work toward changes in muscle strength, muscle size, or muscle endurance, which can be measured. Measured progress is evidence that your weight training effort is effective, and it serves as a motivating influence to continue.

Suggested Lifetime Fitness Weight Training Programs

The following training programs have worked well for adults as lifetime weight training programs:

(1 × 15–20): 1 set of 15 to 20 repetitions

(1 × 8–12)

(2 × 10)

(3 × 10)

(3 × 8)

(3 × 6)

(3 × 10, 8, 6)

(3 × 20, 10, 5)

(DeLorme 3 × 10)

The (1 × 15–20) workout is one in which you perform one set of each exercise, attempting to complete 20 repetitions. If you complete all 20 repetitions in good exercise form, the weight on that exercise can be increased for the next training session. You should be able to complete at least 15 good repetitions. If you cannot complete at least 15 repetitions, the weight is too heavy. If you can complete more than 20 repetitions, the weight is too light.

The (1 × 8–12) workout is the same as the previous workout except you should be able to get at least 8 repetitions. If you get more than 12 good strict repetitions, you could increase the resistance for the next training session (progressive overload).

The (2 × 10), (3 × 10), (3 × 8), and (3 × 6) workouts can be performed using the same weight for 2 or 3 sets with a short 1- or 2-minute rest between sets. If you can complete all repetitions in every set, the weight can be increased for the next training session. For example, using the (3 × 8) workout, you might perform the barbell curl using 50 pounds and attempting 8 repetitions in each of 3 sets. When you can complete 8 repetitions in all three sets, you could increase the resistance to 55 pounds for the next training session (progressive overload).

Another option is to add slightly more weight for each set with the last set being your repetition maximum (RM). For example, using the (3 × 8) workout, you might use 40 pounds for your first set, 45 pounds for your second set, and 50 pounds for your third set, with 50 pounds being your 8-RM (8-repetition maximum). For the next training session, you could try 45, 50, and 55 pounds. If you get all 8 repetitions in each set, you could go to 50,

55, and 60 pounds for the next training session (progressive overload)

The (3 × 10, 8, 6) workout consists of three sets. The first set is 10 repetitions, the second set is 8 repetitions, and the third set is 6 repetitions. Each set is done with a heavier weight.

The (3 × 20, 10, 5) workout includes three sets of each exercise. The first set is 20 repetitions. Twenty repetitions will provide a good warm-up as well as a stimulus for developing muscle endurance. The second set is 10 repetitions. Ten repetitions will provide some stimulus for an increase in muscle endurance, some stimulus for an increase in muscle size, and some stimulus for an increase in muscle strength. The third set is 5 repetitions. The first two sets should have the muscles and joints warmed up and ready for this heavier load. Five repetitions with a heavy resistance will provide a stimulus for an increase in muscle strength.

The (DeLorme 3 × 10) workout consists of three sets of 10 repetitions.

First set: 10 reps with 50% of your 10-RM

Second set: 10 reps with 75% of your 10-RM

Third set: 10 reps with 100% of your 10-RM

The first set of 10 repetitions should be performed with 50% of your 10-repetition maximum (10-RM). Your 10-RM is the heaviest weight that you can lift 10 times. The second set of 10 repetitions should be performed with 75% of your 10-RM. The third set should be performed with 100% of your 10-RM.

When you can complete 10 repetitions in the third set, the weight used in that set is increased for the next training session, and the first two sets are adjusted according to this new 10-RM. You should be able to get at least 8 repetitions in the last set with the new weight. Keep working with that weight until you can get 10 good repetitions. Then the weight is increased again. You should never get fewer than 6 good repetitions in the last set. If you cannot get at least 6 good repetitions, you have increased the weight too much and should reduce the weight for the next training session.

The DeLorme method is fast and easy on weight-stack machines but involves quite a bit of weight changing when using barbells, especially when alternating sets with a training partner.

Based on the information presented in this chapter, complete "Planning Your Personal Weight Training Program," using the chart provided at the end of this chapter.

A Simple Home Training Program for Busy People

This is a simple training program that you can do at home. It takes very little time and very little money, but it can make a very big difference. The only equipment required is a set of two adjustable-weight dumbbells and a flat exercise bench. These items often appear inexpensively at garage sales. The eight exercises are as follows:

Chest: dumbbell bench press
Back: one-dumbbell rowing
Shoulders: seated dumbbell lateral raise
Arms (biceps): seated dumbbell arm curls
Arms (triceps): seated one-dumbbell triceps extension
Hips and thighs: dumbbell lunges
Lower leg: one-dumbbell calf raise
Abdominals: Crunches

Perform all these exercises every other day. If it takes 1 minute to perform each exercise and 1 minute between each exercise to rest and change the weight for the next exercise, you would complete this workout in 16 minutes. Realistically, plan on 20 minutes, especially as the resistance increases. For better total fitness results, perform 20 minutes of continuous aerobic exercise on nonlifting days. Convenient, inexpensive aerobic exercises include walking, jogging, and stair-stepping at home.

If this is still too time-consuming, split the weight training program by performing the upper-body exercises one day (the first five exercises) and the

Dumbbell Bench Press

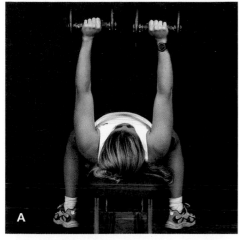

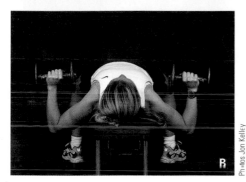

Photos Jon Kelley

One-Dumbbell Rowing

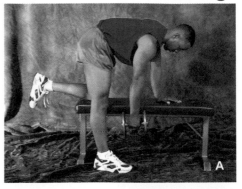

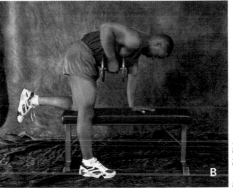

Photos Eric Risberg

Dumbbell Lateral Raise

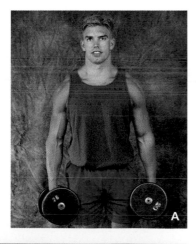

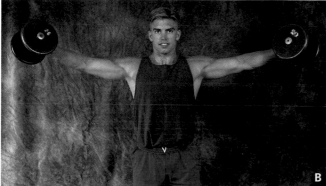

Photos Eric Risberg

Seated Dumbbell Curl

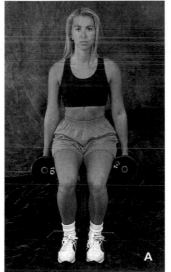

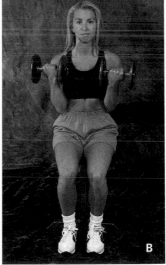

Photos Eric Risberg

One-Dumbbell Triceps Extension

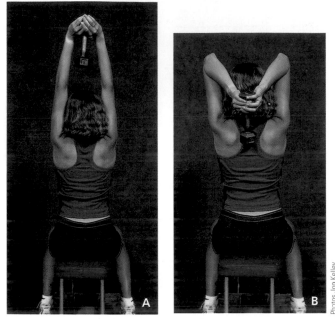

Photos Jon Kelley

Dumbbell Lunges

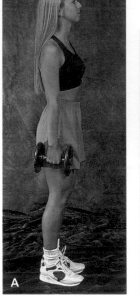
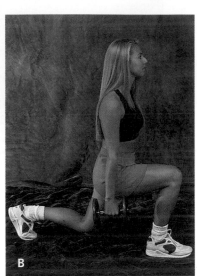

Photos Eric Risberg

One-Dumbbell Calf Raise

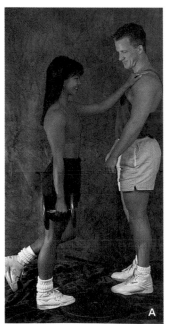
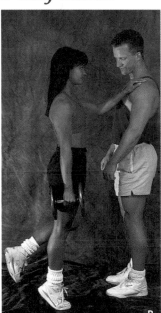

Photos Eric Risberg

Crunches

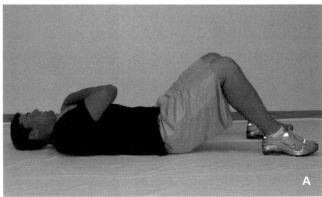

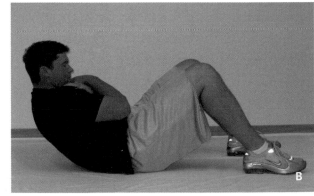

Photos James Hesson

Name _____ Section _____

Planning Your Personal Weight Training Program

Directions

1. Read Chapter 16, "Planning Your Personal Weight Training Program."
2. Plan a weight training program that is consistent with your goals from Chapter 15.
3. Refer to the exercise chapters for general body part and specific exercises.
4. Refer to Chapter 16 for resistance, repetitions, sets, rest, and frequency.

Chapters 8–13   **Table 16.1**

General Body Part	Specific Exercise	Resistance % of 1-RM	Repetitions	Sets	Rest Interval	Frequency Days/wk.
Chest						
Back						
Shoulders						
Arms						
Legs						
Abs						
Back Extension						

Name _____ Section _____

Planning Your Personal Weight Training Program

Directions

1. Read Chapter 16, "Planning Your Personal Weight Training Program."

2. Plan a weight training program that is consistent with your goals from Chapter 15.

3. Refer to the exercise chapters for general body part and specific exercises.

4. Refer to Chapter 16 for resistance, repetitions, sets, rest, and frequency.

General Body Part	Specific Exercise	Resistance % of 1-RM	Repetitions	Sets	Rest Interval	Frequency Days/wk.

lower-body exercises the next day (the last three exercises). The upper-body workout takes approximately 10 minutes every other day, and the lower-body workout takes about 6 minutes every other day.

During the first month, perform one set of 20 reps of each exercise. The second month perform one set of 15 reps of each exercise. The third month perform one set of 12 reps of each exercise. After 3 months, you might want to just maintain on this workout, or you might want to try some of the other set and rep combinations suggested in this chapter.

Time Management

Time management is really self-management. You can't manage time; however, you can manage yourself and your use of time. You need to take control and manage your life. Everyone is equal when it comes to time. Each person gets 24 hours each day and 168 hours each week.

You can invest, spend, or waste your time. Once time passes, it is gone forever. That part of your life is over. You can't go back; you can only go forward. Where are you going with your time and with your life?

First Assignment

Carry a time schedule with you for 1 week and jot down what you really do each hour of each day. You might learn a lot about yourself and your use of your time.

Second Assignment

Plan your time. Failing to plan is planning to fail. There are too many things for one lifespan to buy. You cannot have and do everything. You must choose exactly what you want and invest your time to get it. You need to budget enough time to "buy" your most important goals.

Your time schedule is a plan to help you get what you want. You will be a product of what you do with the time you have. If you want to "be different," you need to "do different."

Many readers of this book are university students, so the following example will be for them. However, if you are not a student, you can adapt it to your situation. This is your time and your life, and you must decide how to budget and schedule your time to get what you want.

1. *Decide* what time you will get up each day. Fill it in on the time schedule at the end of this chapter. Then, fill in 1-hour time blocks for 24 hours.

2. *Plan* your time schedule around your fixed commitments. (Classes, employment, exercise, eating, and sleeping.) Other fixed commitments will depend on your priorities. Sleep is very important for your health, exercise progress, and learning. Most people need about 8 hours each night to recover physically, mentally, and emotionally. If you can't get everything done in 16 hours a day, maybe you're trying to do too much. Go to your time schedule and fill in your fixed-time commitments.

3. *Plan* the exact time of day and length of time you will exercise. Individuals who have exercise goals, an exercise plan, and a scheduled exercise time are better about sticking with regular exercise. Also, those who exercise first thing in the morning are more likely to stick with it. Later in the day there are more interruptions, and your energy level might decrease. Also, exercise first thing in the morning increases your metabolic rate for several hours following exercise. This means you should be more alert and burn more calories. Still, there is much to be said for exercising at the end of your "workday" as a way to relax and socialize. The best time of day to exercise is a time you will do it and a time when you will enjoy it.

4. *Schedule* enough study time for each subject. Most university classes require about 2 hours of study time outside of class for every hour in class. Be precise when you schedule your study time—for example, "Study English" or "Study Weight Training" or "Study Chemistry."

One hour of study immediately after class when the material is fresh in your mind is more effective and efficient than 2 hours later in the week. The 1- and 2-hour free periods between classes are often the most effective times to study.

Change to another subject after 1 or 2 hours on the same subject to maintain your concentration. Plan these study changes into your study schedule. Intermittent study is generally more effective than massed study. That is, 1 hour of study six times a week is more effective than 6 hours of study one time a week. Cramming the night before an exam is a very poor way to learn and a sure sign of poor time management and poor study skills.

5. *Plan* some miscellaneous time. Life never goes exactly as planned. You don't have to schedule every hour of every day. Schedule some miscellaneous time each day and each week to trade for scheduled times that get interrupted to handle emergencies and unexpected things that come up. Plan to study early in your day and relax later in your day. Most students do much better when they study early in the day when they are rested, and relax later in the day when they are tired.

6. *Plan* some relaxation time, some recreation time, some social time, some family time, and some time with friends.

Time	Monday	Tuesday	Wednesday	Thursday	Friday	Saturday	Sunday

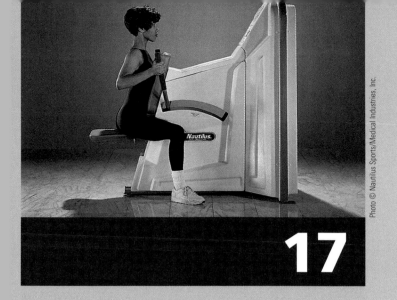

17

Beyond the Basics

Progressive overload is necessary for continued improvement. There are many ways to increase the overload, and some of them are briefly described in this chapter. If overload increases too quickly, your risk of injury increases. Most weight training injuries are the result of trying to do too much too soon. Progressive overload must be applied gradually at a rate that your body can adapt to and recover from.

Progressive Overload

Progressive overload is the basis of all successful weight training programs. The muscles can be overloaded in many ways and depends on all of the following variables:

Which exercises are performed

How many total exercises are performed

How many exercises are performed for each body part

Order in which exercises are performed

Amount of resistance used in each set

Number of repetitions per set

Number of sets per exercise

Amount of rest between sets

Frequency of training sessions

Method of progression

Whether the exercise load is fixed or variable

Whether the total body is exercised in each training session or is divided into a split routine

Exercise intensity

These variables may be changed and combined in a seemingly unlimited number of ways. Some of the more common training programs will be presented to give you an idea of the variety available to you in weight training. All these training programs are different ways to arrive at the same thing: progressive overload.

Beginning weight trainers tend to gain on almost any weight training program. The greatest danger for beginners is overtraining. If you find yourself training very hard, not making any progress, and feeling tired all the time, you are probably overtraining and should try less exercise and more rest.

Humans cannot maintain absolute peak condition for very long—a few weeks at best. Therefore, highly trained advanced weight trainers, competitive lifters, and bodybuilders use periodization, or cycling. They divide the year into periods, or cycles, and then vary their training methods and intensity during the cycles so that they reach their peak condition during their competitive season and hopefully for their most important contest of the year.

Increasing Exercise Intensity

One of the first things that weight trainers try to do as they advance in their training is increase the intensity of their exercise. The following are seven common methods of increasing exercise intensity. All these methods increase your risk of injury, so caution is advised.

Concentric Failure

To reach **concentric failure,** you must perform repetitions until you cannot perform another repetition while maintaining strict exercise form.

Forced Reps

Forced reps are repetitions performed after reaching concentric failure. When you cannot perform another repetition correctly, a spotter assists as little as possible to help you complete 1 or 2 more repetitions.

Negatives

Negatives occur when you lower a heavier weight than you can lift. To perform **negatives,** spotters help you lift a weight and then you lower the weight

by yourself. This advanced training method can result in extreme muscle soreness and is not recommended for beginning weight trainers.

Eccentric Failure

When you perform negatives (lower a weight) until you can no longer control the speed at which you lower the weight, you have reached **eccentric failure.** This is obviously dangerous and is not recommended for anyone.

Cheating

Cheating is the use of other body movements to get past the weakest point in the range of motion. An example of cheating is bouncing a barbell off of your chest and arching your back on the barbell bench press in order to move a heavier weight. While cheating enables you to move a heavier weight, it also increases your risk of injury.

Preexhaustion

Preexhaustion is the use of an isolation exercise for a muscle, followed by a compound exercise for the same muscle. The idea is to work a larger muscle to concentric failure using a single-joint isolation exercise and then force the fatigued muscle to continue working with the assistance of smaller weaker muscles using a multijoint compound exercise. An example is using the dumbbell flye exercise to work the pectoralis major to concentric failure, followed quickly by the barbell bench press to continue working the fatigued muscle with smaller assisting muscles like the triceps, which are used for elbow extension on the barbell bench press.

Postexhaustion

Postexhaustion is the opposite of preexhaustion. The compound exercise is done first, usually to the point of concentric failure, followed quickly by a single-joint isolation exercise for the same major muscle. An example would be the barbell bench press followed by dumbbell flyes.

Periodization, or Training Cycles

Advanced lifters use training cycles, or **periodization,** during which they vary the exercise intensity and volume to reach a peak during their competitive season. The following is a simple example of a training cycle to reach a peak of maximal strength:

5 sets of 10 reps (4 weeks)

4 sets of 5 reps (4 weeks)

3 sets of 3 reps (4 weeks)

2 sets of 1 rep (1 week)

In this periodization model, the total volume of training is reduced, and the resistance is increased with each period of training. This is just a very brief model to quickly illustrate the general idea of periodization. Periodization models can be very complex and entire books are written describing periodization and the theories behind it.

Undulating Periodization

With **undulating periodization,** the training zones are not performed sequentially as in traditional periodization but are varied with each training session. The following is a simple example of one possible undulating periodization model to help you understand the basic concept:

4 sets of 5 reps on Monday

2 sets of 15 reps on Wednesday

3 sets of 10 reps on Friday

The idea is to vary the sets, reps, and resistance with every training session.

Note: Beginning weight trainers do not need to use any of these methods of increasing exercise intensity as long as they are making steady progress. All these methods of increasing exercise intensity also increase your risk of injury. It is your choice. You decide if the risk is worth it, and you accept the responsibility for your decision.

Total Body and Split Routines

Beginners, fitness weight trainers, competitive weight lifters, and advanced bodybuilders typically conduct their training routines differently.

Total Body Routines

Beginners and fitness weight trainers often perform all their weight training exercises during a single training session and repeat this procedure every other day. They exercise the **total body** in each training session.

Split Routines

As weight trainers advance and the total workload increases, many choose to split their exercises, performing part of them one day and the rest of them on another day. One example is the 4-day **split routine** in which half of the exercises are performed on Monday and Thursday and the other half on Tuesday and Friday. An example of a 4 day split is a push–pull routine in which the pushing exercises are performed on Monday and Thursday and the pulling exercises on Tuesday and Friday. Another example is performing the upper body exercises on Monday and Thursday and the lower body exercises on Tuesday and Friday.

Some advanced bodybuilders go to a 6 day split in which they perform about a third of their exercises on Monday and Thursday, a third on Tuesday and Friday, and a third on Wednesday and Saturday. The ultimate split is the blitz routine, in which they exercise only one body part each day.

Fixed Systems

Fixed systems are those in which variables are not changed during a training session, but a variable may be changed for the next training session. There are several types of fixed systems.

Simple Progressive System

A **simple progressive system** involves changing only one variable, such as the resistance. An example is performing one set of 10 reps of an exercise. If 10 reps are completed, the resistance is increased for the next training session.

Double Progressive System

A **double progressive system** calls for changing two variables such as resistance and repetitions. An example is performing one set of 12 reps. If 12 reps are completed, the resistance is increased for the next training session, and the repetitions are decreased to 8. The repetitions are then increased by one each training session until one set of 12 reps is completed with the new resistance. Then the resistance is increased, and the repetitions are decreased again.

One Set to Failure

A variation of the double progressive system is **one set to failure.** In this system, one set of each exercise is performed to the point at which you cannot perform another repetition while maintaining correct exercise technique. A weight is used that causes this concentric failure to occur between 8 and 12 reps. When you complete 12 reps, the weight is increased for the next training session.

Set System

The **set system** requires the lifter to perform more than one set of each exercise. In a fixed system, the repetitions remain the same for each set. One example is 3 sets of 6 reps. When you can complete 6 reps in all 3 sets, the weight is increased for the next training session. This is a good program when you are training with barbells because it reduces the amount of time you spend changing weights.

Circuit System

In a **circuit system,** a series of exercises is performed in a sequence, or circuit, with one exercise at each station. You move from one exercise to the next, performing one set of each exercise until you have completed every exercise in the circuit once. Then the entire circuit may be repeated. The circuit of exercises is usually completed one, two, or three times during a training session.

Circuit training is often used with a large group when time and equipment are limited. This is frequently the case with athletic teams. Circuit training allows a large number of people to get a good workout in a short time.

Aerobic Circuit System

In an **aerobic weight training circuit,** exercises are performed one immediately after the other with no rest between exercises. This is done to keep your heart rate elevated during the entire circuit and thus produce a training effect for your cardiovascular system. An aerobic circuit training program may include an aerobic exercise station between each weight training station.

Super Set System

A **super set** requires performing two exercises in a sequence, followed by a rest interval. Often, opposing muscle groups are exercised in this manner. For example, the first set might be barbell curls for the elbow flexors. The next exercise might be tricep extensions for the elbow extensors. Because these muscles work in opposition to one another, one of them is resting while the other is working. After 1 set of each exercise, there is usually a rest interval before repeating the sequence. This is a good way to reduce training time without reducing the amount of work completed during the training session. It is like a minicircuit.

Examples of Super Set Exercises

Leg Extension and Leg Curl

Overhead Press and Lat Pulldown

Chest Press and Rowing

Ab Crunch and Back Extension

Giant Sets

Giant sets usually involve three to five exercises for the same muscle. One set of each exercise is performed with little or no rest between sets. After all exercises in the sequence have been performed, there is a rest interval before the sequence is repeated.

Example of a Giant Set for Chest

Barbell bench press

Incline dumbbell bench press

Parallel bar dips

Dumbbell flyes

Perform these exercises with no rest between sets. Rest after the last exercise and then repeat the sequence.

Rest–Pause System

The **rest–pause** system has many variations, and here is one: Perform an exercise to the point of temporary muscular failure, hold the weight while the muscle recovers slightly, perform another repetition, pause, do another repetition, and continue until no more repetitions can be performed.

Variable Systems

In **variable systems,** one or more variables are altered during the performance of one exercise.

Pyramid System

In a **pyramid system,** the weight used for each set of an exercise is increased, and the number of repetitions is decreased correspondingly. This allows you to proceed from a light weight to a heavy weight. This system is often used when training for strength. Some weight trainers choose to pyramid up only. Others pyramid up to a heavy weight and then back down again.

Percentage System

The **percentage system** is a variation of the pyramid system. Multiple sets of an exercise are performed at various percentages of your 1-RM for that exercise. The percentages usually start out low in the first set and increase in each of the subsequent sets.

DeLorme System

One good percentage system for beginners and those training for fitness is the **DeLorme system:**

First set: 10 reps at 50% of your 10-RM

Second set: 10 reps at 75% of your 10-RM

Third set: 10 reps at 100% of your 10-RM

Continuous Set System

In the **continuous set system,** or drop set system, start with a weight that you can use to complete a given number of repetitions—for example, 10 reps. When you reach the point at which you can do no more repetitions, your training partner quickly removes a small amount of weight while you continue to hold the bar or stay in position on the machine. As soon as some weight has been removed, the exercise is continued until you cannot do any more repetitions. Once again your training partner removes a small amount of weight. This process continues until you cannot do any more repetitions, even with the lightest weight.

Light-to-Heavy System

The **light-to-heavy system** is a variation of the pyramid and continuous set systems. Start with a light to moderate weight and perform 3 reps. Your training partner quickly adds a small amount of weight. After 3 more repetitions, another weight is added. This process continues until you can perform only 1 rep.

Tonnage System

The resistance and repetitions usually vary in the **tonnage system,** but you keep track of the total pounds lifted during a training session. Each time a weight is lifted, it is multiplied times the number of repetitions completed. For example, a 200-pound weight times 10 repetitions equals 2000 pounds, or 1 ton. The total number of pounds or tons lifted during a training session is added together. Competitive weight

lifters use this system most often. Competitive weight lifters who vary their sets, reps, and resistance with each training session use the tonnage system to keep track of their total training volume.

These are a few of the methods weight trainers have used to apply progressive overload. There are many more and many variations of each of these systems.

Training Equipment

Resistance training equipment includes constant external resistance equipment, variable resistance equipment, and isokinetic equipment.

Constant External Resistance Equipment

Barbells, dumbbells, and some weight-stack equipment have a resistance that is constant. The weight remains the same throughout the exercise. Because of changes in leverage at the joints involved during movement through the full range of motion, this fixed weight is more difficult to lift at some joint angles and easier at others.

With **constant external resistance equipment,** you are limited to the heaviest weight that you can lift through the weakest point in the range of motion. Two basic equipment design approaches have attempted to overcome this limitation: variable resistance equipment and isokinetic equipment.

Variable Resistance Equipment

Some weight-stack equipment has been designed so that, as changes in leverage take place for the working muscles and joints, the exercise machine makes compensating leverage changes. When you are exercising with constant external resistance equipment, once you can get past the weakest point in the range of motion, the rest of the exercise movement is fairly easy. With the compensating leverage change of **variable resis-**

tance equipment, the muscle must continue to work hard throughout the full range of motion. The weight in the stack lifted remains constant, but the leverage change in the machine makes the resistance greater at some joint angles and less at other joint angles. The intent of variable resistance equipment is to keep the muscles fully loaded throughout the full range of motion.

Isokinetic Equipment

Isokinetic equipment offers another solution to keeping the muscle fully loaded throughout the full range of motion. Isokinetic (*iso* = equal; *kinetic* = motion) refers to constant motion or constant speed. True isokinetic exercise equipment limits the speed at which the exercise device will move. Therefore, a muscle can contract at its maximum force from full extension to full contraction without producing acceleration.

Which Type of Exercise Equipment Is the Best?

So far no one particular type of exercise equipment has been proven superior for the development of muscle tissue. Muscles don't know or care what type of exercise equipment is used to provide the resistance, as long as they receive the same overload stimulus. However, keep in mind the principle of specificity. Specificity of training is certainly a consideration when choosing exercise equipment for athletes.

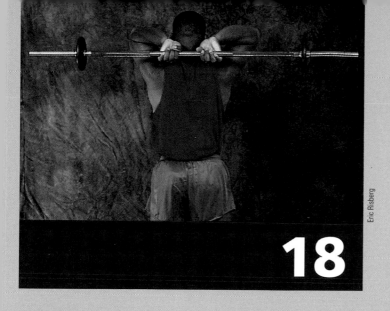

Eric Risberg

18

Weight Training for Life

Anyone can start a weight training program, and many do, but few stick with it. The following are some ideas, strategies, and tips for sticking with your weight training program and getting the results you want.

Transtheoretical Model of Behavior Change

Behavior change is usually a gradual process that involves several stages. Psychologists James Prochaska, John Norcross, and Carlo DiClemente have developed the Transtheoretical Model of Behavior Change, which describes six stages of change.

1. Precontemplation. In this first stage, you are not interested in changing. You may not know you need to change, or you may deny a need for change. If you are in this stage, you might say, "I **don't need or want** a weight training program."

2. Contemplation. In this second stage, you have begun to recognize a need for change, and you are beginning to consider a change. Perhaps you have noticed a loss of strength, vitality, or undesirable changes in your appearance, and you have started thinking about an exercise program to build your strength, regain your vitality, or improve your appearance. If you are in this stage, you could say, "I **might** start a weight training program."

3. Preparation. In the third stage, you are seriously planning to change a behavior within the next month. You might sign up for a weight training class, read a weight training book, join a fitness center, or start looking for a personal trainer. If you are in this stage, you might say, "I **will** start a weight training program this month."

4. Action. In this fourth stage, you have made a commitment and have taken action. If you are in this stage, you might say, "I **do** have a planned weight training program, and I lift weights at a regular time and place."

5. Maintenance. In the fifth stage, you have maintained your behavior change for a long time. If you are in this stage, you might say, "I **have been** weight training on a regular basis for the last five years."

6. Adoption. In the sixth stage, you have adopted a positive behavior and it has become part of your lifestyle. If you are in this stage, you might say, "I **am** a weight trainer." The behavior has become a regular part of your current lifestyle and your identity.

Relapse is when the person returns to an old behavior. Relapse may set in at any level after precontemplation. Occasionally you will miss a workout or a week of weight training—everyone does. Life can be planned, but you need to be flexible enough to adapt to changes that occur. Sometimes in life, you must bend with the wind, but you need to spring back as soon as the wind lets up a bit.

Relapse is *not* failure. It is human. We can strive for perfection but must accept excellence. *Weight training for life* is a continuous process of starting over and adapting to change.

Changing your behavior is one of the most difficult challenges in life. It is stressful. If you change to healthier behaviors, however, you will become more resilient and better able to cope with change and stress. It is easier not to lift weights, but it is better to overcome resistance.

It is easier not to learn, but it is better to learn. The easy path does not lead to the top of the mountain. You cannot reach your full potential by taking the easy path. You cannot improve yourself or your life by staying on the easy path.

Tips for Sticking with It

The following are ideas that will help you adhere to your weight training program and get the results you want.

Motivation

Needs and wants motivate behavior. The depth of your desire to meet a need or want determines the strength of your motivation. Once you reach your goal, it loses its power to motivate. After all, now you have what you want. To be motivated to continue weight training, you need to set new goals. The new goal could be further improvement, or it could be to maintain what you have achieved.

Enjoyment

Enjoyment is extremely important in sticking with your weight training program. Most people seek pleasure and avoid pain. We find time for the activities we enjoy and find excuses to avoid the activities that are difficult and painful for us.

If you enjoy weight training, you will find a way to do it on a regular basis. If you design a personal weight training program for yourself that is a long, boring, terrible, painful experience, you will find excuses to avoid it.

Different people find enjoyment or satisfaction in exercise in different ways. Some of the things that bring enjoyment to weight training are improvement, challenge, excitement, relaxation, competition, and social interaction.

Importance

Regular lifelong weight trainers have a common belief that weight training is good for them. A lot of evidence supports that belief. If you haven't read the evidence yet, maybe you should start now. To continue regular weight training, you must believe that the benefits you receive from your program are worth the time, effort, energy, and money you put into it.

Priority

To stick with your program, you must place a high priority on it. Build it into your schedule and stick with the time you have set for training. You will always be able to find other things you could do during that time, but don't allow those other things to replace your training time.

Time

We all have the same amount of time each year, each month, each week, and each day. Some people make time for exercise, and some claim they don't have time to exercise. Surveys have indicated that the average American watches 3 to 4 hours of television each day, and yet these same people claim they don't have time to exercise. Clearly, for most people, exercise is not a question of time but, instead, one of priorities. Schedule your weight training time and stick with it.

Record

Improvement is a powerful motivator for most people. Write down the relevant information from each weight training session. These records will provide visible evidence of your improvement and of your ability to stick with a weight training program.

Reward

Regular weight trainers get a sense of satisfaction, an intrinsic reward, from regular exercise sessions. As a beginner, however, you may benefit from extrinsic rewards. You might want to promise yourself something for reaching a goal you have set for yourself. Of course, it should be a healthy reward, and you should get it only when you reach your goal.

Knowledge

The more you learn about weight training, the more you understand the benefits, the more you know about correct technique, the more you know about designing programs, the more likely you are to continue. Most people want to be good at something. If you are willing to learn and to stick with your training, you can become good at weight training.

Social Interaction

Some people enjoy the social benefits of weight training. They like to exercise with a friend or a small group. They enjoy the new friends who they meet when they are weight training. If you meet people while you are weight training, you instantly have something in common and a topic of conversation with them.

Support

Share your new weight training goals and your new weight training program with people who you know will be supportive. Get support from as many people as you can. Once you tell a large number of people that you are going to do something, it becomes harder to quit and easier to continue.

Identity

When you become a regular weight trainer, it becomes a part of your identity. Once it is a part of who you are and what you do, it is easier to stick with it and harder to quit. Friends and family no longer ask if you are going to work out, they know when you are going to work out.

Place

If you like the place where you exercise, you will want to go there. If you don't like the place where you do your weight training, you will not want to go there. Therefore, you should find or create a pleasant place to do your weight training.

Convenience

If weight training is too inconvenient, you are more likely to quit, so you should seek ways to make weight training as convenient as possible. Identify the obstacles to regular weight training and begin to eliminate them one by one.

Instruction

Most people get satisfaction from doing something well. Getting good instruction whenever you start a new activity is usually an excellent investment of your time and money. Excellent instruction gets you past the awkward beginner stage more quickly. Getting good weight training instruction when you are beginning will get you past the beginner stage more quickly and will help you avoid mistakes.

Variety

Weight training programs offer a wide variety of options. Some people prefer a highly structured routine that almost never changes. They like to do the same exercises in the same order at the same time on the same days for years. Others like to do something different during every training session. Most people are somewhere in-between. They like to follow an exercise plan for 6 weeks, 8 weeks, 12 weeks, or some other block of time and then change their program for the next block of time. You need to determine what works best for you— what keeps the training fun and interesting for you.

Fitness

If you can stick with a weight training program long enough to reach a fitness level that you are proud of, you are more likely to continue to train for the rest of your life. It is much easier to maintain a higher level of fitness than it is to get there in the first place.

Success

You can learn to set reasonable goals. You can learn to plan weight training programs to reach your goals. You can learn to stick with your weight training program. You can improve your fitness level. You can achieve success through weight training.

Appearance

In our society, appearance is important. We are bombarded by daily messages— from movies, television, and advertising—that looking good is important. Although it is okay to want to improve your appearance and look good, self-worship is not attractive. One of the most effective and efficient ways to improve your appearance is weight training.

Image

Your body image is how you see yourself. Most people have a subconscious drive to maintain a body that is consistent with their body image. This does not mean a perfect body. Even if we could come to some general agreement of what the perfect body would look like, training for perfection is unrealistic and unattainable. Instead, we should train for a healthy body image. Although you cannot change your genetic body type, you can make the most of what you have.

Regularity

The greatest benefits of weight training come from making regular training a lifelong habit. Losers weight train too hard for a short time, then quit, and do nothing for a long time. They may start again, but they generally train too hard again for a short time and then quit again. Winners are consistent in their training. They generally train at a more moderate pace and design programs that are realistic, lifetime weight training programs. Will you choose to be a winner or a loser?

Habit

Your body adapts gradually to weight training. Healthy weight training is a healthy lifestyle habit much like brushing your teeth. It is most effective if it is done regularly and continuously as a part of your routine of living. Good habits bring good results. Bad habits bring bad results. We make our habits; then our habits make us.

Weight Training for Life

If you don't take care of your body, where will you live? Do you know people who take better care of their house or car than their body? You may live in many houses and drive many cars in your lifetime, but you get only one body to live in for your entire life. Take good care of it by *weight training for life*.

Place a checkmark by the tips for sticking with it that you believe will help you the most with weight training for life.

___ Motivation	___ Place
___ Enjoyment	___ Convenience
___ Importance	___ Instruction
___ Priority	___ Variety
___ Time	___ Fitness
___ Record	___ Success
___ Reward	___ Appearance
___ Knowledge	___ Image
___ Social Interaction	___ Regularity
___ Support	___ Habit
___ Identity	

References and Suggested Readings

Aaberg, E. *Resistance Training Instruction.* Champaign, IL: Human Kinetics, 1999.

Allsen, P. E. *Strength Training: Beginners, Bodybuilders, and Athletes,* 3rd ed. Dubuque, IA: Kendall/Hunt Publishing, 2003.

Alter, M. J. *Sport Stretch,* 2nd ed. Champaign, IL: Human Kinetics, 1998.

American College of Sports Medicine. "Exercise and Physical Activity for Older Adults." *Medicine and Science in Sports & Exercise* 30, no. 6 (1998): 992–1008.

American College of Sports Medicine. "The Recommended Quantity and Quality of Exercise for Developing and Maintaining Cardiovascular and Muscular Fitness, and Flexibility in Healthy Adults." *Medicine and Science in Sports & Exercise* 30, no. 6 (1998): 975–991.

American College of Sports Medicine. "Appropriate Intervention Strategies for Weight Loss and Prevention of Weight Regain for Adults." *Medicine and Science in Sports & Exercise* 33, no. 12 (2001): 2145–2156.

American College of Sports Medicine. "Progression Models in Resistance Training for Healthy Adults." *Medicine and Science in Sports & Exercise* 34, no. 2 (2002): 364–380.

American College of Sports Medicine. *ACSM's Guidelines for Exercise Testing and Prescription,* 7th ed. Philadelphia: Lippincott/Williams & Wilkins, 2005.

American College of Sports Medicine. *ACSM's Resource Manual for Guidelines for Exercise Testing and Prescription,* 5th ed. Philadelphia: Lippincott/Williams & Wilkins, 2005.

Anderson, B., E. Burke, and B. Pearl. *Getting in Shape,* 2nd ed. Bolinas, CA: Shelter Publications, 2002.

Antonio, J., and J. R. Stout. *Supplements for Strength-Power Athletes.* Champaign, IL: Human Kinetics, 2002.

Baechle, T. R., and B. R. Groves. *Weight Training: Steps to Success,* 2nd ed. Champaign, IL: Human Kinetics, 1998.

Baechle, T. R., and R. W. Earle. *Essentials of Strength Training and Conditioning,* 2nd ed. Champaign, IL: Human Kinetics, 2000.

Baechle, T. R., and R. W. Earle. *Fitness Weight Training,* 2nd ed. Champaign, IL: Human Kinetics, 2005.

Bennett, J. *The Basics of Weight Training Workbook.* Boston: Allyn & Bacon, 1995.

Bompa, T., M. Di Pasquale, and L. Cornacchia. *Serious Strength Training,* 2nd ed. Champaign, IL: Human Kinetics, 2003.

Boyle, M. A. *Personal Nutrition,* 4th ed. Belmont, CA: Wadsworth/Thomson Learning, 2001.

Briggs, D. *16 Weeks to Weight Training Success!* Dubuque, IA: Kendall/Hunt, 2003.

Brzycki, M. *A Practical Approach to Strength Training,* 3rd ed. Indianapolis: Masters Press, 1995.

Cissik, J. M. *The Basics of Strength Training.* New York: McGraw-Hill Higher Education, 1998.

Cole, S., and T. Seabourne. *Athletic Abs.* Champaign, IL: Human Kinetics, 2003.

Cook, B., and G. W. Stewart. *Strength Basics: Your Guide to Resistance Training for Health and Optimal Performance.* Champaign, IL: Human Kinetics, 1996.

Delavier, F. *Strength Training Anatomy.* Champaign, IL: Human Kinetics, 2001.

Delavier, F. *Women's Strength Training Anatomy.* Champaign, IL: Human Kinetics, 2003.

Earle, R. W., and T. R. Baechle. *Essentials of Personal Training.* Champaign, IL: Human Kinetics, 2004.

Evans, N. *Men's Body Sculpting.* Champaign, IL: Human Kinetics, 2004.

Fahey, T. *Super Fitness for Sports, Conditioning, and Health.* Needham Heights, MA: Allyn & Bacon, 2000.

Fahey, T. *Basic Weight Training for Men and Women,* 4th ed. New York: McGraw-Hill, 2004.

Fahey, T., and G. Hutchinson. *Weight Training for Women.* Mountain View, CA: Mayfield, 1992.

Faigenbaum, A., and W. Westcott. *Strength and Power for Young Athletes.* Champaign, IL: Human Kinetics, 2000.

Field, R. W., and S. O. Roberts. *Weight Training.* Boston: WCB/McGraw-Hill, 1999.

Fleck, S. J., and W. J. Kraemer. *Designing Resistance Training Programs,* 3rd ed. Champaign, IL: Human Kinetics, 2004.

Goldenberg, L., and P. Twist. *Strength Ball Training.* Champaign, IL: Human Kinetics, 2002.

Hales, D. *An Invitation to Fitness and Wellness.* Belmont, CA: Wadsworth/Thomson Learning, 2001.

Hales, D. *An Invitation to Health,* 11th ed. Belmont, CA: Wadsworth/Thomson Learning, 2004.

Hansen, J. *Natural Bodybuilding.* Champaign, IL: Human Kinetics, 2005.

Hoeger, W. W. K., and S. A. Hoeger, *Principles and Labs for Fitness and Wellness,* 7th ed. Belmont, CA: Wadsworth/Thompson Learning, 2004.

Hoeger, W. W. K., L. W., Turner, and B. Q. Hafen. *Guidelines for a Healthy Lifestyle,* 3rd ed. Belmont, CA: Wadsworth/Thomson Learning, 2002.

Howley, E. T., and B. D. Franks. *Health Fitness Instructor's Handbook,* 4th ed. Champaign, IL: Human Kinetics, 2003.

Incledon, L. *Strength Training for Women.* Champaign, IL: Human Kinetics, 2005.

Kinakin, K. *Optimal Muscle Training.* Champaign, IL: Human Kinetics, 2004.

Kraemer, W. J., and S. J. Fleck. *Strength Training for Young Athletes,* 2nd ed. Champaign, IL: Human Kinetics, 2005.

Lox, C. L., K. A. Martin, and S. J. Petruzzello. *The Psychology of Exercise: Integrating Theory and Practice.* Scottsdale, AZ: Holcomb Hathaway, 2003.

Moran, G. T., and G. McGlynn. *Dynamics of Strength Training and Conditioning,* 3rd ed. New York: McGraw-Hill Higher Education, 2000.

Newberry, D., K. Kaufman, and J. Baker. *Skills, Drills, & Strategies for Strength Training.* Scottsdale, AZ: Holcomb Hathaway, 2000.

NSCA *Certification Commission. Exercise Technique-Checklist Manual.* Lincoln, NE: NSCA Certification Commission.

O'Connor, B., J., Simmons, and P. O'Shea. *Strength Training Today,* 2nd ed. Belmont, CA: Wadsworth/Thompson Learning, 2000.

Peterson, J. A., C. X. Bryant, and S. L. Peterson. *Strength Training for Women.* Champaign, IL: Human Kinetics, 1995.

Roberts, S. O., and D. Pillarella. *Developing Strength in Children: A Comprehensive Guide.* Reston, VA: American Alliance for Health, Physical Education, Recreation and Dance, 1996.

Sandler, D. *Weight Training Fundamentals.* Champaign, IL: Human Kinetics, 2003.

Schoenfeld, B. *Sculpting Her Body Perfect,* 2nd ed. Champaign, IL: Human Kinetics, 2003.

Smith, C., and D. Jones. *Conditioning and Weight Training,* 3rd ed. Dubuque, IA: Kendall/Hunt, 2001.

Tesch, P. *Target Bodybuilding.* Champaign, IL: Human Kinetics, 1999.

Trestrail, R. T. *Weight Training: A Practical Approach to Total Fitness.* Dubuque, IA: Kendall/Hunt, 1999.

Westcott, W. *Building Strength and Stamina,* 2nd ed. Champaign, IL: Human Kinetics, 2003.

Westcott, W., and T. R. Baechle. *Strength Training Past 50.* Champaign, IL: Human Kinetics, 1998.

Westcott, W. L., and T. R. Baechle. *Strength Training for Seniors.* Champaign, IL: Human Kinetics, 1999.

Whitmarsh, B. *Mind & Muscle.* Champaign, IL: Human Kinetics, 2001.

Index